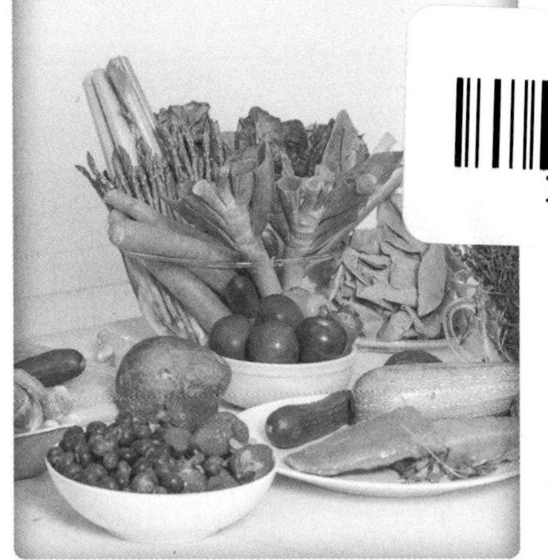

Contents

Foreword vii

Introduction
My Philosophy on Food, Nutrition, and Diet: People Who Love Food Are the Best 1

Chapter 1
Food Feelings: How Emotions, Habits, and Attitude Shape Your Food Story 11

Chapter 2
Gut Feelings: The Five Aspects of Optimal Health 23

Chapter 3
Get to Know Your Bio-Individuality: Seven Tests to Consider 55

Chapter 4
Break Up with the Foods That Don't Love You 83

Chapter 5
Love the Foods That Love You Back:
Food Groups, Superfoods, and Antioxidants 105

Chapter 6
Food Rules for Living Life to the Fullest:
Dining Out, at Home, and While Traveling 153

Chapter 7
Feed Your Hormone Balance:
A Woman's Guide to Nutrition Cycle 183

Chapter 8
Feed Your Hunger for Health:
Protocols for Specific Health Conditions 209

Chapter 9
Foodie Kitchen Essentials, Food Shopping List,
and Recipes 245

References 315

About the Author 343

Praise for THE FOODIE DIET

"Ella Davar, RD, brings together the best of functional nutrition and practical wisdom. *The Foodie Diet* is a clear, actionable guide to using food as medicine, focusing on anti-inflammatory, nutrient-dense choices and personalized strategies rooted in diagnostics. A valuable resource for anyone serious about long-term health and healing."

—**Mark Hyman. MD,** co-founder and chief medical officer, Function Health, and #1 *New York Times* bestselling author of *Young Forever*

"Ella Davar has written a book that finally makes food simple again. *The Foodie Diet* is about eating real, unprocessed food—animals, plants, and everything nature intended—without fear or confusion. It's a practical guide for anyone who wants more energy, better health, and a longer life, starting with what's on their plate."

—**Paul Saladino, MD,** author of *The Carnivore Code*

"Ella Davar's *The Foodie Diet* brings clarity to the connection between health, metabolism, and longevity. With science-based insights and practical strategies, she translates complex nutrition research into daily habits that support healthspan and resilience—an approach that reflects the principles we study at the Buck Institute for Research on Aging."

—**Eric Verdin, MD,** president and CEO, Buck Institute for Research on Aging

"*The Foodie Diet* offers a refreshing, nutrition-forward approach to longevity. Ella Davar emphasizes the importance of balanced nutrition with adequate protein and fiber at every meal—principles that support muscle, metabolic health, and resilience over a lifetime. This book provides busy individuals with practical, actionable strategies to optimize both healthspan, musclespan, and performance."

—**Gabrielle Lyon, DO,** board-certified family physician and *New York Times* bestselling author of *Forever Strong*

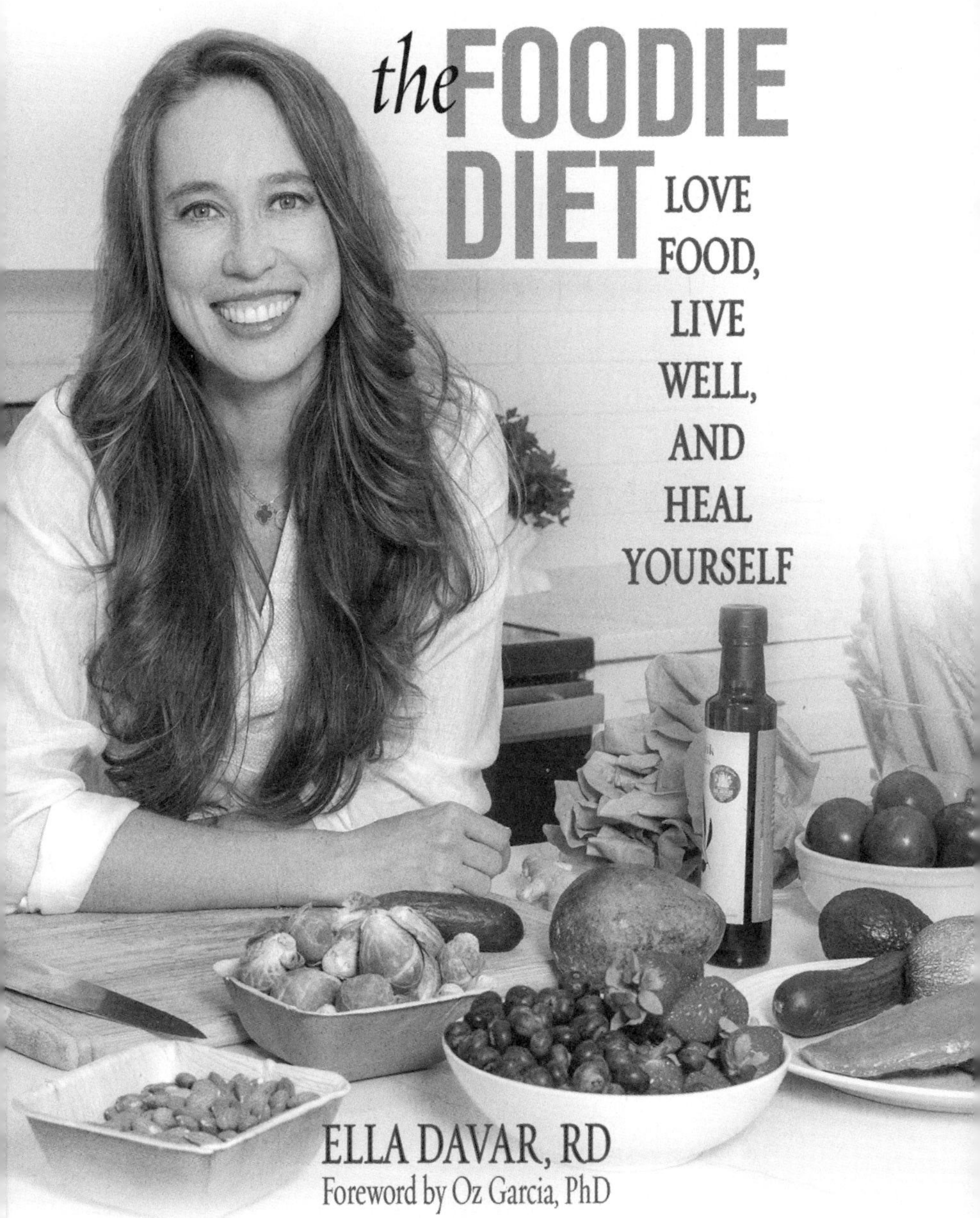

the FOODIE DIET

LOVE FOOD, LIVE WELL, AND HEAL YOURSELF

ELLA DAVAR, RD

Foreword by Oz Garcia, PhD

Health Communications, Inc.
Mt. Pleasant, South Carolina

www.hcibooks.com

Library of Congress Cataloging-in-Publication Data
is available through the Library of Congress.

ISBN-13: 978-07573-2544-1 (Paperback)
ISBN-10: 07573-2544-0 (Paperback)
ISBN-13: 978-07573-2545-8 (ePub)
ISBN-10: 07573-2545-9 (ePub)

Publisher: Health Communications, Inc.
1240 Winnowing Way, Suite 102
Mt. Pleasant, SC 29466

Cover photo by Dmitrii Bezrukov
Cover, interior design, and formatting by Larissa Hise Henoch

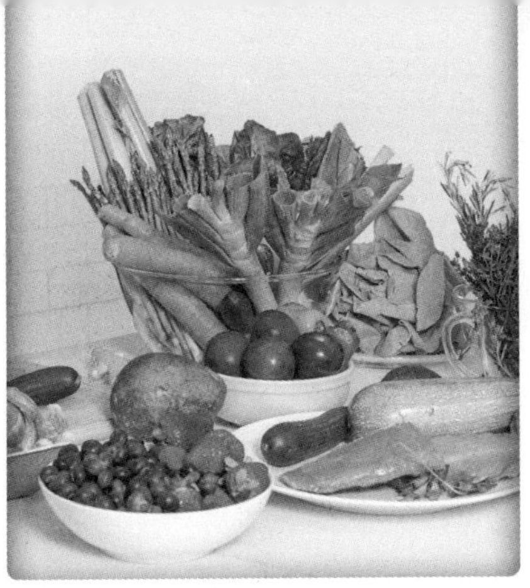

Foreword

In my forty years as a nutritionist, I've seen the wellness world evolve in remarkable ways. From the early days of green juice pioneers and biohacking entrepreneurs to the global movement around gut health, we've witnessed a shift—from symptom management to true root-cause healing. And yet, despite all the supplements, protocols, and lab testing, one thing remains irrefutable: food is still the most powerful medicine we have.

That's what makes *The Foodie Diet* so refreshing. In a world saturated with trends, labels, and rigid diet ideologies, Ella Davar brings us back to what matters most—joy, optimal nourishment, and self-awareness. *This isn't a book about restriction; it's a guide for liberation.* A path to reclaiming the wisdom of your body and rebuilding a sustainable relationship with food through science and soul.

Ella has a rare gift. She blends evidence-based nutrition and longevity science with deep emotional intelligence. I know this not just as a peer in the wellness space, but personally. After a long battle with long COVID, it was Ella who came into my home with healing hands and a heartfelt presence. She didn't arrive with supplements or clinical protocols—though she could have. Instead, she made me bone broth, meatballs with vegetables, and classic, soul-supportive meals rooted in traditional cooking and anti-inflammatory principles. What she offered was far deeper than nutrition. It was care, presence, and food that fed more than my cells—it nourished my spirit.

The Foodie Diet is her first major work, and it couldn't come at a more crucial time. As someone who has spent decades helping others optimize longevity, I can say with full confidence that Ella is defining how the next generation will be educated about food and wellness. She's a rising voice in our field who has already been featured on the cover of *The Wall Street Journal* as a leader in the longevity movement. Her work is rooted in science, but grounded in real-life nourishment—food that connects, heals, and empowers.

This book invites you to explore food not just as fuel or function, but as a mirror to your habits, emotions, and personal history. Ella brings you into that inquiry with compassion, offering frameworks and protocols, yes—but also the emotional context that most nutrition books leave out. That alone makes this required reading.

Whether you're a practitioner, a curious foodie, or someone simply trying to find your footing again after years of conflicting advice, *The Foodie Diet* is your reset. Look inside. This book will help you remember how to love food again—and how to let food love you back.

—**Oz Garcia, PhD,** renowned neuro-nutritionist
and life extension specialist, author of *After Covid: Optimize Your Health in a Changing World*

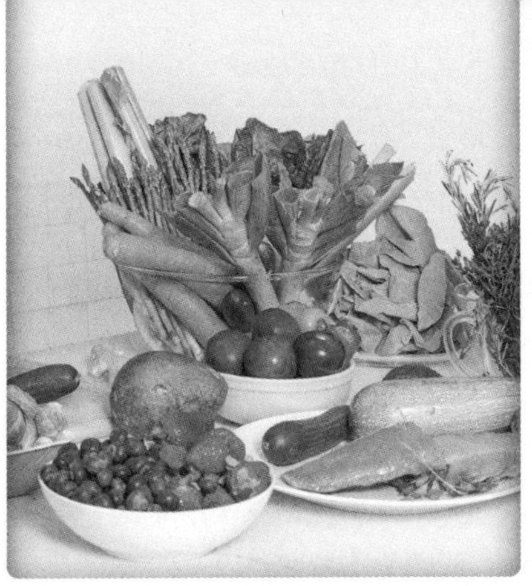

Introduction

My Philosophy on Food, Nutrition, and Diet

I love food. I plan my day and travel around eating at the best places and sharing food with loved ones. Always have, always will. When other people tell me they "forget to eat," I stare at them in bewilderment. Food isn't just sustenance for me—it's a passion, my art, and my work, and ultimately what transformed my entire life. I love food so much that I devoted my life to becoming a food expert, leaving behind a successful Wall Street career to pursue my true calling.

If you've picked up this book, chances are you're confused about what the right diet is for you. You may also be frustrated because you love food and you just want to enjoy it. I get it—I love food too! In fact, I probably love it even more than you. I love it so much that

I devoted my life to becoming a food expert. If you are a busy, ambitious, and health-conscious urban professional, biohacker, foodie, and a woman interested in natural beauty and wellness, this book is for you.

In this book, you will find a refreshing and relatable "nondiet," a love-based approach to nourishment that lets you savor every bite and cut through the noise of the fad diets and restrictive weight-loss advice. I am here to tell you that you don't need any more books about keto, veganism, or the paleo diet. Trends aren't trending anymore as more of us choose to politely disagree and quiet down the noise. My goal is to show you how functional nutrition, longevity science, and personalized medicine—the main areas of focus in this book—can come together to add joy back into your meals no matter what health issues you might be facing.

I also wrote this book because I wanted to share my story. I know what it's like to feel stuck and confused, sick and hopeless, and to try really hard to fix things but still feel like you are spinning your wheels. Ever since I was a little girl, I've struggled with progressive vision loss and inflammatory gut conditions despite being raised on all-natural foods. I grew up in Russia, and my family ate a very healthy diet, but it wasn't because my parents were particularly cautious or health conscious. It was simply the natural lifestyle we lived. My parents didn't have the money to buy manufactured products—in Russia they are imported and thus more expensive—so Coca-Cola was reserved for holidays, a rare treat. Instead, my family was self-sufficient and resourceful, growing most of our food in my grandparents' garden near the town where I was born. I grew up eating a high-protein diet with locally sourced plants—whole, organic, and nontoxic—all homegrown.

Yet by the age of fourteen, I developed an inflammatory stomach condition called gastritis. *How*, you might ask, *could this happen to someone raised on such healthy foods?* It certainly wasn't because I ate junk food—most of my meals were made from scratch. That's how I learned to cook, and it's why I've included an entire chapter in this book dedicated to easy, delicious recipes you can make at home.

The root cause of my condition wasn't food; it was internalized stress and emotions. My father was a strict and demanding man who wanted me to succeed in life and believed the way to do this was by instilling discipline and hard work. These characteristics, in and of themselves, are not bad—but he held me to impossibly high standards. As a young child, I coped by bottling up my emotions, which is never healthy. I internalized a lot of stress from constant pressure and unexpressed negative emotions. I was diagnosed with gastritis due to persistent stomach pain and GI imbalance, and by the age of fifteen, I was taking so much medication that I vividly remember sitting in front of a pile of tinctures and pills, trying to memorize the protocol of which ones to take on an empty stomach, which after meals, and which before bed. I burst into tears, feeling so sick, overwhelmed, and hopeless. At that moment, I realized I was taking more medication than my grandmother, and I felt sick and lonely because most people in my family were very physically fit.

As a dietitian, I now see similar struggles in my clients. Many of their health issues aren't solely food related but also stem from their inner critic, born from their emotionally unstable upbringing. They are often far too hard on themselves, trapped in a heightened perception of stress and self-criticism. I understand this deeply because I've lived it.

This is why I begin this book with a chapter focused on emotional health and how our feelings can manifest as physical ailments. My story is a testament to the profound connection between our mind and body, and my goal is to empower you to address not only what's on your plate but also what's in your heart and mind.

I struggled with health problems for years after I grew up and left home, especially while working on Wall Street in New York City in a highly demanding work environment. I was so confused about what to eat that I saw every health expert and tried every diet under the sun: Keto. Paleo. Vegan. Ayurvedic. Macrobiotic. Juice cleansing. Intermittent fasting. Fortunately, there was a dietitian who finally changed my life by changing my relationship with food. I started to listen to my body, invested in testing, and became a *you-tarian*. I created a personalized diet that actually worked for me. I learned to listen to my body to determine my own nutritional needs and develop a personalized nutrition plan that worked for my body and for my lifestyle. It was transformational. No more diets, no more deprivation, no more "experts" telling me what to eat and what not to eat. I was able to solve all my health problems and feel better than I ever thought possible. Moreover, I still love food and mindfully indulge on occasion (including some incredible meals at world-class restaurants).

I went on to invest a lot of time, money, and energy into studying nutrition science, human biochemistry, and medical nutrition therapy, going deep into scientific research while becoming a licensed nutrition and food expert and getting educated at multiple universities, academies, and institutes—so you don't have to. *The Foodie Diet* shares all my top-secret hacks and tricks of the trade that I've been dishing out to my global roster of high-achieving, ambitious clients in Miami, New York City, Paris, and beyond.

Coming to terms with my inner food obsession, learning what

my body thrives on, and using some handy nutrition science hacks allows my clients and me to enjoy a healthy lifestyle and have some dolce vita too. That's why I wrote this book. I don't want anyone to have to choose between being a foodie and healing themselves with whole foods. I believe—and know—that you can have your cake and eat it too (forgive the lame joke, but it's true). Yes, this is possible, and this, my friend, is the goal of becoming what I call a *professional foodie*: someone who eats their way to a healthier life and does it with enjoyment and love.

Diet trends are constantly changing, but the real wisdom of balanced nutrition hasn't changed in over one hundred years. We're going to mine the tried-and-true rules of balanced nutrition in a way that you can easily apply to your life, with maximum pleasure and nourishment and minimum restriction. Some of the advice I share will be familiar, but I think you'll find that the approach overall is a bit different than what you may have already tried. In addition to arming you with the essential foundation of healing the gut and building a diet full of anti-inflammatory foods, I'm going to guide you on an inner journey to empower your relationship with food. That means discovering your food story, learning *why* you eat what you eat, uncovering the emotions behind your cravings, and finally, getting to know your own body: what it loves and thrives on and what it hates and would be better off without. You'll learn how to turn every meal, whether it's a chef's tasting menu or a healthy snack on the go, into an act of mindfulness, love, and self-care.

The core of the Foodie Diet approach is developing a personalized nutrition plan based *on loving the foods that love you back.* I'm going to encourage you to drop the diet labels ("I'm vegan/keto/pescatarian/fill-in-the-blank-here") and embrace the liberation that comes with simply being a *you-tarian: a person who knows how to eat what is best for them at any given time*, whether it's a steak or a cake, a green juice or a cup of coffee (organic and fair trade, please!). As people who love food, we want to learn to identify and love the foods that our *body* loves, which is sometimes different from what we crave or think of as healthy. Loving food this way is a different kind of love, one that's more meaningful and sustainable—like a healthy, fulfilling partnership rather than a series of bad dates with people you know aren't good for you.

The Foodie Diet is about falling in love with the foods that love you back and developing a relationship with food that is exciting, pleasurable, abundant, nourishing, and creative. Like any good relationship, it brings joy, supports you in challenging times, and enriches your life in countless ways. Let's get started.

There is disagreement among experts in health care on whether we should be vegan or carnivore. I would like to offer a different idea by giving you a glimpse at what the future of the wellness field looks like and empower you to get to know your body and design a diet that works for you and your love of food. I am going to offer you an easy way to learn about hormones, gut health, genetics, methylation, and seasonality, which help my clients create diet rules that fit their lifestyles.

Before I became a registered dietitian, like many other young women, I struggled with dieting and conflicting health advice in the wellness world. After years of dieting and trying many different diet approaches, I became a dietitian and nutrition expert to empower women to connect with their bodies.

It took me years to come to terms with my love for food. I tried to deny it, suppress it, avoid it, and substitute it with love for results and discipline. Once I accepted my true self instead of trying to be like everyone else, I felt liberated—and you will too. I wrote this book for young women trying their hardest to find the food that is right for them.

I begin by covering your relationship with your body. Physical health is where it all starts, and love of food is a combination that has been hard to navigate and harmonize for most women throughout their lives. The conditions were planted in your childhood. When you were a child, how did you use food? Some children learn that it is the only thing they can control in their lives or the only thing that brings them pleasure.

I wrote this book for all of us to thrive together while empowering one another to live fully and embrace our greatest potential. This is for the younger version of myself—and for everyone out there feeling confused about what to eat or which diet to follow in pursuit of better health, energy, and confidence, one day at a time. Thank you to everyone who inspired me to create this book. I see you, I feel you. I've been there too.

Pro Tip from a Dietitian

What I've learned over the last twelve years of working in the wellness industry is that your health condition and optimal wellness are not going to change by taking one pill or supplement, doing one special workout routine, or drinking one $25 smoothie shake elixir. It will come down to hard work—a lot of understanding, learning, and daily commitment to choosing what's best for you. While you are the one to put it all into practice, I have done the groundwork and wrote this book to simplify the process for you.

People Who Love Food Are the Best People

During my medical dietetic training in New York hospitals, I repeatedly heard doctors and healthcare providers label patients as "lazy," assuming they would inevitably make bad food decisions. This insulting, pessimistic view infuriated me. As I looked around, I didn't see people trying to be unhealthy. Instead, I saw people being crushed by a system that makes processed food convenient and cheap while placing healthy, organic produce out of reach for many.

This frustration fueled my mission. I invested years studying nutrition science, diving deep into health and longevity research, and getting educated at multiple universities and institutes. What I discovered transformed my understanding: Healing your body doesn't mean giving up the joy of eating. You can nourish yourself *and* love every bite. Real food can be both medicine and indulgence—no need to pick sides.

When we talk about healing ourselves and regaining health, what we really mean is cellular health—specifically, the health of our mitochondria, the tiny powerhouses in our cells responsible for energy production. This is where real healing begins, not with the latest trending diet or Netflix documentary. Real transformation comes from understanding your unique body and making daily choices that honor both your health and your love of food.

This book isn't about choosing between being a plant lover or an animal lover. It's about understanding your unique body and giving it what it needs to thrive. I'm going to share with you the framework I've developed through years of clinical practice and personal experience. You'll learn about functional nutrition, longevity science, and personalized medicine—the real foundations of lasting health.

Your body is a complex network of intricately connected systems, far smarter than any diet trend or documentary. It's time to start trusting and listening to its innate wisdom.

Let's rediscover the art of food, the joy of eating while healing yourself and your family, one mindful bite at a time.

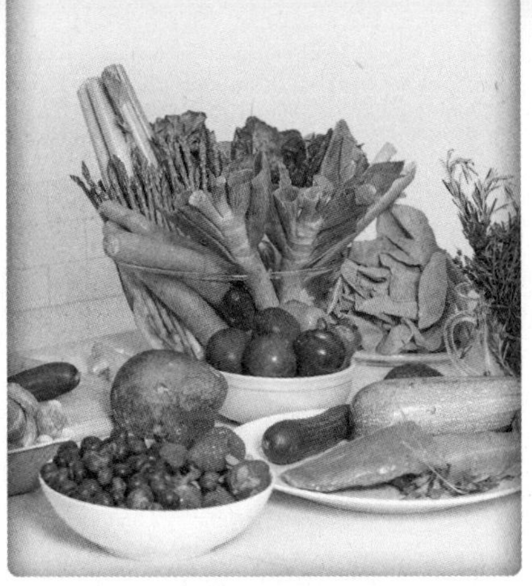

Chapter 1

Food Feelings: How Emotions, Habits, and Attitude Shape Your Food Story

Before we dive into what to eat, let's take a step back and look at something more fundamental: your relationship with food—your big *why*. This journey begins not with what's on your plate but with *what's in your heart and mind,* what fuels your desires and goals.

Most people come to my office asking for nutrition advice and meal plans. They begin their understanding of food intake by trying to learn the facts on how to gain control over the right food groups, calorie count, and nutrient density. Most of us have a basic understanding of healthy eating, which is not enough. When it comes to compliance and our daily habits, the challenge isn't about lack of knowledge or willpower—that's a myth. Instead, we come up with emotional reasoning: *We've got to live a little. Life is too short. This food takes me back to my childhood.* We struggle to maintain healthy habits in the face of peer pressure, guilt, emotional voids, and addictions. I want to address the big elephant in the room with this first chapter by answering this question:

Why do we do what we do when we know what we know?

I love food, and I believe you should, too. But loving food and having a healthy relationship with it are two different things. Throughout my years as a functional medicine dietitian, I've seen how our deepest emotions become entangled with our eating habits, creating patterns that can either nourish or destroy us.

My own journey taught me this lesson firsthand. Despite my passion for food, I once struggled with my choices. I constantly felt bloated and tried every diet imaginable to get leaner. I used food to soothe my anxiety, reward my achievements, and find a sense of control. I'd swing between strict discipline and sugar binges, caught in a cycle that many of my clients find familiar. It wasn't until I addressed the emotional roots of my eating habits with food therapy that I finally found balance, embracing what I now call the *80/20 rule*: eating clean and mindfully 80 percent of the time while allowing for conscious indulgence the other 20 percent.

Your relationship with food is like any other relationship in your life. It can be a healthy, supportive partnership that makes you feel like you can take over the world or a toxic cycle that drains your energy and makes you feel awful—but you keep going back out of habit. Just like in romantic relationships, we bring our past with us to the table, quite literally.

The Childhood Connection

From our very first moments, food becomes intertwined with love, care, nourishment, and survival. Whether through breast-feeding or bottle-feeding, our earliest experiences with food literally wire our nervous system. This is why I always ask about childhood diets before working with clients. These early patterns tell me crucial information about what we're facing.

As we grow up, food becomes the first thing we are able to control, especially when we step into our teenage years and try to assert ourselves in the world. Life is complicated, and our relationships with other people are often unstable, so most things around us are outside our control. That's why children are picky: A picky eater is someone who can assert themselves in the world by saying no to things, maybe for the first time ever, and this eventually becomes part of their character. How parents respond to this natural assertion through food—whether with punishment, negotiation, or respect—shapes how we'll approach self-advocacy and pleasure throughout our lives. This pattern shows up later in life when some people become afraid of being inconvenient in restaurants by vocalizing their preferences and asking for what they want. I have to teach my clients how to do that, especially in group settings. Some people just prefer to roll with the vibes and become a product of the environment rather than advocate for their needs.

Take sugar addiction, for example. I often trace it back to childhood habits of eating sweet treats to cope with a stressful home environment. That bowl of Lucky Charms becomes more than breakfast —it's emotional comfort when Mom and Dad aren't providing it.

One of my clients repeatedly asked about the best food to consume when he woke up hungry in the middle of the night. I provided all the best high-protein and fiber options and ways to prevent nighttime hunger. Eventually, during an inner healing meditation, I asked about his childhood relationship with food. He revealed that he felt so lonely in his family that he always ate in his bed. This core memory had solidified in his brain—he should be eating in bed. Once we acknowledged the loneliness within him, he was able to stop eating and fill himself with self-compassion in moments of loneliness instead of trying to soothe emotions with food.

Function over Flavor

During my dietetic residency study-abroad program at New York University, our group traveled to Israel. In a Bedouin village on the Egyptian border, local women welcomed us by making traditional bread, their hands expertly working the dough before baking it in hot ashes—a technique passed down through generations. While most of us gathered around, mesmerized by the process and the heavenly aroma, several of my fellow dietetic students hung back. They sat alone, methodically eating premeasured portions of gluten-free and dairy-free options of cucumbers, eggs, and nuts from plastic containers they'd packed at the hotel. Right there, in the middle of this rich cultural food experience, these future nutrition professionals were so focused on controlling their intake that they missed a once-in-a-lifetime chance to experience food as culture, connection, joy, and a huge learning opportunity.

I see this pattern intensify with clients who've been traumatized by health diagnoses—whether it's Lyme disease, small intestinal bacterial overgrowth (SIBO), or irritable bowel syndrome (IBS). Their diagnosis becomes their identity, leading to obsessive control over dietary limitations. They become overly attached to their condition, avoiding entire food groups and obsessively tracking every bite. While this hypervigilance might produce the desired test results, it often creates a new problem: the stress of constant control. The perception of stress around food can be as harmful as eating the "wrong" foods.

These clients forget that joy is a nutrient also. They remove pleasure from the equation, seeing it as frivolous or dangerous rather than essential to healing. But here's what I tell them: Your relationship with food is as important as the food itself. When we strip away all enjoyment in the name of health, we create an unsustainable pattern that can actually hinder our recovery.

One of my clients came to me proudly identifying as a strict vegetarian for five years, believing it was the healthiest and most environmentally responsible choice. She'd built her entire social identity around this dietary choice, following all the vegan influencers, joining online communities, and even starting a blog about her lifestyle. But beneath this carefully constructed identity, she was struggling. During business trips, she'd spend hours researching restaurants that could accommodate her restrictions, often missing out on team dinners and local experiences. When visiting her family, she'd bring her own food rather than share traditional home-cooked meals with loved ones, creating a sense of control and health benefits at the cost of isolation and loneliness.

Through our work together, she realized how her rigid vegetarian identity had become a shield—a way to feel in control and gain validation from others. As we worked on nutrient-dense meal plans and a healthy mindset for hormonal balance during menstrual changes, we explored more flexible approaches. She discovered the concept of being a flexitarian, someone who primarily follows plant-based eating but allows for adaptability. This became her bridge to true food freedom. Eventually, she embraced becoming a *you-tarian*, listening to her body's needs rather than following external rules.

Now she enjoys family meals again, learning and cooking new recipes with her loved ones, trying local specialties when traveling, and, most importantly, feeling liberated from the need to define herself through dietary labels and rules. She's learned that true health isn't about conforming to others' expectations or seeking validation through food choices. It's about honoring your body's wisdom and adapting to life's various situations with grace.

Comfort Eating or Filling Up the Emotional Void?

Let's talk about what nobody wants to discuss: comfort eating to fill an emotional void. Whether it's stress, loneliness, boredom, or anxiety, using food as an emotional bandage is incredibly common. My working clients tend to complain about this pattern: after laboring extra hard to earn a living or a paycheck, or pushing for that raise, the only joy at the end of the day becomes that extra dessert in front of the TV. It's a way to comfort physical exhaustion and soothe the emotional void left by a day of avoiding our feelings. High-sugar foods, in particular, influence brain chemistry by triggering dopamine release, which can temporarily help us numb feelings we'd rather not face.

Studies show that workplace stress significantly impacts our eating patterns, with over 70 percent of professionals reporting stress-eating behaviors. Eventually, this stress creates a double burden—we're not just dealing with the stress of our jobs but also the guilt that comes after emotional eating. Many of my clients get caught in this cycle: stress at work → comfort eating → guilt about eating → more stress → more eating. Breaking this cycle isn't about willpower; *it's about creating new pathways to process our emotions.* When one of my clients started taking actual lunch breaks to eat mindfully with colleagues and taking three deep breaths before the meal (more on that later) instead of working through lunch and bingeing later, not only did her eating habits improve, but her work performance did too, as she found a reason to smile by creating joyful moments during her lunch break. *We must learn to feel our feelings in real time rather than stuffing them down with food.*

In our society today, overeating, overindulging, ordering too much food, eating junk food, and being obese are socially acceptable. It is challenging and sometimes lonely to choose the best for yourself. As part of my career education, I worked on a research project at Mount Sinai in New York, where I educated parents and low-income communities in the Bronx about healthy habits. I saw firsthand how difficult it is to choose a healthy lifestyle in neighborhoods where food deserts are the norm—no grocery stores, just mini-marts, fast-food chains, and cheap treats—and when all their peers and friends are eating what is advertised to them every day. Unfortunately, cauliflower and broccoli farmers don't have huge marketing budgets to advertise to us, and making healthy choices becomes our responsibility as we mature and serve as role models for younger population groups.

So how do we keep from comfort eating to fulfill emotional voids? My advice: *Diversify your sources of pleasure and non-food-related joy.* When food becomes your only joy after a long day or when you're unable to prioritize your well-being, overindulgence—especially in sugar, alcohol, and oversized restaurant portions—feels like a natural escape. Instead, schedule dance breaks, find small daily joys, say a kind word to yourself (or use affirmations), and create multiple pathways to happiness that don't involve eating.

Think about it now: *What feeds your soul? What makes you feel happy to be alive?* And how can you do more of that?

Breaking the Pattern

Every time you reach for food, pause and ask yourself:

- Am I hungry, or am I feeling something I don't want to feel, like boredom or a lack of inspiration?
- Have I done something today to bring me joy?
- What can I feed my soul with today? For some of us, it is creating beauty; for others, it is connecting heart to heart with our loved ones. Even a hug is sometimes better than a snack to give us the energy to keep going!

These simple questions begin the process of rewiring those hardwired food habits. When you eat trigger foods, your brain releases dopamine—the feel-good neurotransmitter—reinforcing the habit. But here's the empowering part: You can rewire your brain to make healthier choices feel just as rewarding. Healthy eating is not about deprivation; it's about retraining your brain to seek foods that truly nourish you.

Mind-Body Unity

Let's talk about mindset and why it is so important for successful weight loss and that energetic vitality and lightness in the body that most of my clients are seeking.

Your body hears everything you tell yourself inside your head: *You and your body are one.* This concept transforms everything for my clients seeking change. As my mentor used to say, you can't hate yourself into a version you'll love.

One heartbreaking pattern I see repeatedly in my office is clients who come in speaking so harshly about themselves. They're doing everything right 80 or 90 percent of the time, but they absolutely torture themselves over that 10 to 20 percent of perceived failure. Instead of celebrating their consistent healthy habits, they fixate on that one dessert, that one missed workout, that one bad meal. They come to me looking for someone to berate them, to give them an even stricter plan, to fix what they see as broken within themselves.

But in my programs, I do the opposite. I help them switch their mindset to notice all the good things they've built and done for themselves because my mentor was correct: *You can't hate yourself into a version you'll love*. When we shift our focus from punishment to appreciation, something remarkable happens: Those problem behaviors often resolve themselves naturally, without the need for more rigid rules or restrictions.

The number of negative stories my clients come into the office with—*whoa!* Sometimes it makes me want to stop my clients and ask them, "How did you learn to talk to yourself in such a harsh and unkind way? Who spoke to you like that in your childhood?"

The biochemistry inside our bodies shifts with our thoughts. When we're stressed, cortisol increases, affecting appetite and cravings. When we're optimistic, serotonin flows, helping to regulate mood and appetite.

Pro Tip from a Dietitian

It's absolutely normal to experience body weight fluctuations with your hormonal cycle. Even models get bloated before their periods. That's why I keep pants in a couple of sizes—depending on where I am in my cycle—and encourage my clients to do the same. Choose to feel good in your body, whatever day of the month it is.

The Evolution of Our Relationship with Food

Here's another thought about food feelings. Many of us grow up with certain eating habits, and it's often not until we reach our forties that we start to experience any issues. When those issues arise and can no longer be explained away or ignored, my clients find themselves throwing their hands up in the air, asking me why they've developed prediabetes or dysbiosis. *Why?* they wonder. *I've been eating this way since my childhood.* Yet that way of eating no longer works for them.

Here's something nobody tells you: Your body's "warranty" typically expires around age thirty-five. The truth is that when you take care of things, they last! That's why developing an attitude of looking at food as a medicine as we grow up and using it as a tool to give us a healthy metabolism is an essential part of becoming an adult.

The high-sugar, processed-food diet that carried you through your teens and twenties won't serve you forever. It's not just about your metabolism slowing down. It's about insulin sensitivity and cellular health.

When insulin sensitivity starts to decrease after years of eating high-carb foods like cereals, breads, bagels, snacks, and sugary drinks, weight loss becomes more challenging. Weight gain isn't about a "sluggish metabolism"—it's about your body's changing needs and its ability to process what you feed it.

Moving Forward

The path to healing your relationship with food starts with acceptance. It's okay to love food. It's healthy to seek nourishment, and it's also your responsibility to learn about healthy choices that you can start incorporating on a daily basis to create better outcomes for yourself and your family. Begin by asking yourself,

- How do I see my body right now?
- Do I speak to myself as I would to a dear friend?
- If I truly love myself, what would I choose to eat today?

Just because you grew up eating only certain foods doesn't mean you must (or should!) continue that way. After years of working with clients, I've seen people go from saying, "I hate cauliflower," or "I need to have my cookie in the afternoon," to telling me, "I actually don't mind broccoli now," and "I can't believe I used to eat that—now it's cloyingly sweet."

Challenge yourself to an experiment, and see how your taste buds change if you start introducing healthy habits. Try a new vegetable every week, or experiment with new recipes. You might be surprised at how your preferences evolve! Do a sugar detox, or if that sounds like too much, start by consuming fewer sugary treats.

How do you feel about bitter foods like herbs that are good for you and your liver? There are so many ways—big and small—to improve your relationship with the foods you eat, and I can't wait to share those with you in the rest of this book.

Let's move forward together in creating a relationship with food that serves both your body and your soul.

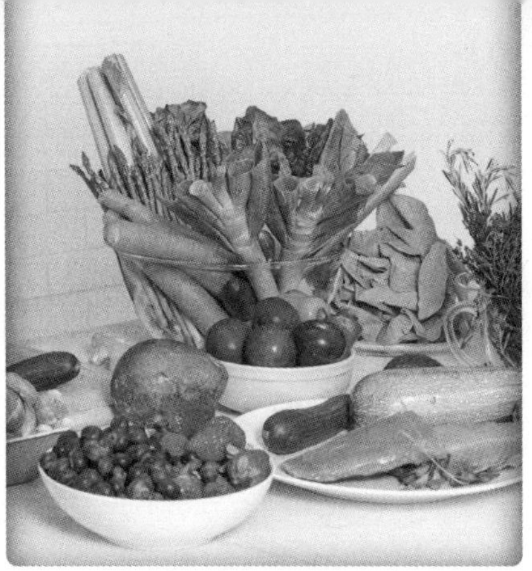

Chapter 2

Gut Feelings: The Five Aspects of Optimal Health

Let's talk about food and what happens to it when we eat it. You've probably heard the oversimplified statement, "You are what you eat." It's actually true, but a lot of processes go on inside our body from the moment we take a bite of our favorite piece of cake and enjoy the taste of it in our mouth until we see it in the toilet bowl again. Most of us rarely stop to consider what happens to our food after we swallow. It's easy to take digestion for granted, as if it's a background process that runs on autopilot, requiring no thought or attention.

However, the body signals us with symptoms like lack of energy, sluggishness, and a slow metabolism. We reach for something *external* to help us fix things, but instead, I'm inviting you to look for *the root cause within*!

After you swallow your food, it hits the stomach and ends up in your intestines for the next eighteen to twenty-four hours. This is where the magic happens. At this point, that piece of cake is no longer cake; it is more of a chyme (a semiliquid mixture of partially digested food and digestive enzymes) that contributes to your gut microbiome makeup. The microbiome is your inner ecosystem, comprising trillions of diverse live bacterial microorganisms and cultures, such as fungi and yeast in your digestive tract.

Everything you eat gets fermented, digested, broken down into nutrients, and then absorbed into your bloodstream to create neurotransmitters and hormones, which affect how you feel. The gut microbiome has become one of the hottest topics in health, and for good reason—it impacts everything from digestion to mood, immunity, and even brain function. Gut health wasn't always taken seriously in the scientific community. I recall a time when most scientists and health researchers would dismiss it with comments like, "Take it to the health food store," implying it wasn't grounded in real science.

Thankfully, those days are behind us. Advances in science have shed light on just how critical the gut microbiome is to overall health. Researchers now understand that gut bacteria play a central role in regulating the immune system, and treatments once considered unconventional—like fecal transplants—are gaining traction as potential solutions for immune conditions and other health challenges. This shift in awareness reflects the undeniable connection between a healthy gut and a healthy body, backed by groundbreaking scientific developments.

Some of us struggle with fatigue, low energy, bloating, indigestion, and skin issues like acne and eczema, and the root cause for all of them is an imbalance of gut microbes. Bad bacteria overgrowth, yeast like candida, or parasites and parasitic infections in the intestines can create those nagging symptoms.

When there's inflammation in the gut, we often feel it in our brain as well—this is called "neuroinflammation." Why? Because the gut and brain are directly connected through the gut-brain axis (GBA), primarily via the vagus nerve—a major communication highway that runs from the brainstem to the gut, regulating digestion, mood, heart rate, and immune responses. Neuroinflammation is linked to stress, anxiety, mood, and even energy levels.

- Do you feel bloated after eating? Are you tired and unable to lose weight?
- Are you eating foods that support your gut microbiome—or ones that might be disrupting it?
- Are you including anti-inflammatory foods in your meals each day, or are you missing those opportunities to nourish your body?

The **gut-brain axis** is the connection between the brain, gut, and microbiome and its potential to profoundly influence our health.

The **vagus nerve** is the body's superhighway, carrying information between the brain and the internal organs and controlling the body's response in times of rest and relaxation.

Every human body is like a garden. Within this garden, our gut is the fertile soil from which everything grows. The health and nutrient density of our soil determines whether it thrives or withers. It's up to us to nurture and care for ourselves—starting with the gut—so our lives can grow abundantly. The more we enrich our soil with nutritious foods, the more bountiful the fruits of our labor—which are optimal metabolism and higher chances of longevity. Whether in business, family life, or creative pursuits, if you're struggling with disease, poor energy and focus, or chronic feelings of anxiety and depression, you need to look at the state of your soil. That means creating a strong foundation of gut health.

By the end of this chapter, my goal is to show you that the health of your gut is the foundation of pretty much everything you want in life. Energy. Clarity. Motivation. Beauty. Well-being. Sexiness and pleasure. (I'm not kidding! Research shows that an imbalanced gut can reduce sex drive and sexual attractiveness.) As you'll learn, gut health affects all the major functions of the body, from digestion and neurotransmitters and hormones to mental health and energy levels. That's why optimizing gut health, which begins with food and ends with breath, is one of the core pillars of the Foodie Diet.

Optimal gut health begins with food and ends with breath.

Gut Health for Foodies

If the promise of improved health isn't motivation enough, there's another *big* reason all foodies should care about gut health: The state of your gut is largely what determines what foods you can and cannot tolerate. With a healthy gut, you can enjoy a wide range of foods with maximum benefit and minimal ill effects. You've heard the expression that you are what you eat. Yes—but more specifically, you are what you digest! The bacteria living in your GI tract—the gut flora or microbiome—help your small intestine break down nutrients for better absorption. Your GI tract is truly fascinating and worth attending to closely. Poor gut health leads to poor digestion and nutrient absorption and also contributes to food allergies, intolerances, and sensitivities. If you can't digest things like gluten, dairy, or soy, you probably have some level of gut imbalance. The good news is that healing the gut fixes the sensitivities, meaning you can enjoy more foods without harming your health or feeling like crap.

Many of my clients who eat organic and exercise regularly still find themselves bloated or struggling with allergies, autoimmune conditions, poor energy, and low-grade anxiety and depression. The answer you have been looking for might be in your gut microbiome.

The Gut-Brain Connection

Your gut is often called the "second brain," and for good reason. Before becoming a dietitian, it was hard for me to grasp how our microbiomes are so intricately connected to our brains. The enteric nervous system (ENS) in the gut contains 500 million neurons—five times as many as in the spinal cord. These neurons don't just control gut muscle movements and enzyme secretions that fuel digestion; they communicate directly with your brain, influencing everything from mood to memory.

Let me share what I've learned through clinical practice: When clients come to me with anxiety or mood issues, we often start by healing their gut. This isn't just theory. I've witnessed remarkable transformations in my clients' mental well-being when we focus on restoring their gut health. The microbiome-mood connection is so powerful that I now consider mental health support a crucial part of any gut-healing protocol.

Think of your gut as a constant conversation with your brain. Every time you eat, you're not just feeding yourself—you're feeding trillions of microorganisms that produce neurotransmitters affecting how you think and feel. This is why I'm passionate about teaching that true mental wellness often begins on your plate.

Up to 95 percent of serotonin, the feel-good hormone responsible for happiness and emotional well-being, is produced in the gut. Research published in *Frontiers in Psychology* highlights this connection, explaining why people with depression, often linked to low serotonin levels, frequently experience gastrointestinal (GI) issues like IBS or abdominal discomfort. Similarly, conditions like IBS and leaky gut are strongly associated with stress, anxiety, and depression, further underscoring the profound relationship between gut health and mental health.

The root cause of many symptoms starts in the gut. Whether your gut is stressed, toxic, dysbiotic, autoimmune, or gastric, identifying your gut type using comprehensive stool testing is the first step toward healing your digestion and optimizing metabolism. As a dietitian, I've seen how this single test can transform treatment approaches. What fascinates me most is how our gut bacteria directly impact our emotional well-being, explaining why low serotonin levels seen in depression and anxiety so often correlate with GI issues. Understanding this connection has revolutionized how I approach both digestive and mental health in my practice.

If you want to improve serotonin production, stabilize your mood, and boost energy, what you eat matters. Prebiotic-rich foods like onions, garlic, and asparagus feed the beneficial bacteria in your gut. Fermented foods such as sauerkraut, kimchi, and yogurt introduce healthy probiotics that diversify your microbiome. Tryptophan-rich foods like salmon, turkey, and eggs supply the amino acids necessary for serotonin production.

Up to 80 percent of your immune system and 90 percent of the neurotransmitters responsible for mood stability are located in your gut. If your gut isn't healthy, your immune system and emotional well-being will struggle. By understanding your gut makeup and prioritizing gut-healthy foods daily, you can positively transform multiple aspects of your life—from mood and energy to digestion and immunity. Your gut truly holds the key to how you feel, think, and function every day.

Gut-Skin Connection: How Your Microbiome Impacts Your Skin

Your skin often reflects what's happening in your gut—because the skin is not just a surface. Your skin is a vital organ that responds to internal imbalances. The gut-skin connection is a fascinating and important pathway that directly links the balance of your gut microbiome to the health and appearance of your skin. When your gut is thriving, it supports glowing, resilient skin. But when the gut microbiome becomes imbalanced—a state known as "dysbiosis"—it can trigger systemic inflammation and immune dysregulation, which often manifest on the skin as acne, eczema, or rosacea. In the case of rosacea, dysbiosis may exacerbate vascular sensitivity and inflammatory pathways, worsening flare-ups and skin reactivity. Over time, this chronic inflammation can also contribute to premature skin aging and the development of fine lines and wrinkles.

Think of it this way: The gut is your body's main nutrient-processing hub. If your gut isn't functioning properly, it impacts how well your body absorbs essential nutrients, including those that keep your skin healthy, like amino acids and vitamin C, which are critical for collagen production. Collagen is the structural protein that keeps your skin firm, elastic, and wrinkle-free. When your gut is off-kilter, your body struggles to produce enough collagen, which can lead to fine lines and sagging skin—effects that may appear prematurely, even before the natural decline in collagen that typically begins around age twenty-five to thirty.

Gut inflammation is another major player here. Chronic inflammation in the gut often spills over into the bloodstream, increasing systemic inflammation. This has been directly linked to skin conditions like rosacea, eczema, and even acne. Research shows that when the gut barrier is compromised—a condition often called "leaky gut"—toxins and inflammatory compounds can escape into the bloodstream, creating a cascade of reactions that show up on your skin.

What's fascinating is how much your gut bacteria do to support your skin. For example, when you eat fiber-rich foods, your gut bacteria ferment that fiber into short-chain fatty acids (SCFAs). SCFAs, such as butyrate, play a key role in reducing inflammation and supporting the skin's barrier function, which helps lock in moisture and protect against environmental damage. A happy microbiome equals hydrated, glowing skin.

It's not just inflammation and collagen. Dysbiosis can trigger hormonal shifts and inflammation that lead to acne breakouts. Studies have shown that restoring gut balance through probiotics and prebiotics can significantly improve these conditions by calming inflammation and enhancing the skin's natural defenses.

So, what can you do? First, focus on feeding your microbiome. Fiber-rich, prebiotic foods like garlic, onions, and artichokes are a great place to start. They fuel the beneficial bacteria in your gut that produce SCFAs, which help reduce inflammation and support healthy skin. Probiotics are also key; fermented foods like yogurt, sauerkraut, and kimchi introduce beneficial bacteria that restore balance and protect your skin from the inside out.

If sagging skin or wrinkles are a concern, boosting collagen production is essential. Make sure your diet includes vitamin C–rich foods like oranges, bell peppers, and strawberries, which support collagen synthesis. Zinc, found in pumpkin seeds, sesame seeds, cashews, and pine nuts, is a key nutrient that supports skin repair and renewal. And don't underestimate the importance of hydration—water keeps your skin plump and elastic while helping your gut absorb and process nutrients efficiently.

Your skin's health isn't only about what you put on it; it's about what you feed your gut. The gut-skin axis is a powerful reminder that glowing, resilient skin starts from within.

Pro Tip from a Dietitian

If you want radiant skin, focus on gut health first. Eat a variety of fiber-rich and prebiotic foods daily, add fermented options for probiotics, and include collagen-boosting nutrients like vitamin C and zinc in your meals. Also take time to manage stress. Chronic stress can disrupt your gut and, in turn, your skin. A healthy gut is the foundation for skin that not only looks great but also feels great.

As a gut health nutritionist, I can't stress enough how vital a healthy gut is for overall well-being and longevity. The gut is at the center of so many things—if it's not happy, the rest of your body won't be either! Symptoms like bloating, brain fog, fatigue, or skin issues can all point to increased intestinal permeability that causes a gut imbalance or leaky gut.

Your gut microbiome plays a pivotal role in nearly every aspect of your health. Here are some reasons why it's so crucial:

1. **Diverse microbiome for disease prevention.** A diverse gut microbiome can significantly reduce your risk of chronic diseases such as obesity and diabetes. For example, studies have shown that individuals with high microbial diversity have a reduced risk of developing metabolic conditions like type 2 diabetes and cardiovascular disease.
2. **Inflammation reduction.** Chronic inflammation is a major driver of aging and age-related diseases. A healthy gut helps reduce systemic inflammation by maintaining a balanced population of beneficial bacteria. This microbial balance prevents the overgrowth of harmful bacteria that can trigger immune activation and inflammatory responses. According to research conducted by the National Institute of Environmental Health Sciences, this gut-mediated regulation of inflammation plays a key role in promoting longevity and may reduce the risk of neurodegenerative conditions, including Alzheimer's disease and other forms of dementia.
3. **Immune system support.** A balanced microbiome enhances your immune response, making your body more efficient at fighting off infections. An imbalanced gut, on the other hand, can weaken your immune system, making you more susceptible to illnesses.
4. **Enhanced nutrient absorption.** Your gut is responsible for absorbing the nutrients your body needs to function

optimally. A healthy gut helps break down and absorb essential vitamins, minerals, and other nutrients, providing the building blocks for energy, tissue repair, and overall health. Poor gut health can lead to nutrient deficiencies, impacting your energy levels and immune function.

5. **Metabolic health regulation.** A well-balanced gut microbiome helps regulate metabolism, preventing obesity and type 2 diabetes.
6. **Mental health connection.** The gut-brain axis is a powerful bidirectional communication pathway. A healthy gut microbiome plays a critical role in producing key neurotransmitters like serotonin and dopamine, which directly influence mood, stress regulation, and cognitive function. According to research from institutions such as the National Institute of Mental Health, this gut-brain interaction helps reduce the risk of mental health conditions such as anxiety and depression, and may even influence the development of neurodegenerative diseases, including Alzheimer's and other forms of dementia.
7. **Hormone balance.** Your gut microbiome influences the production and regulation of various hormones, including those that manage stress and appetite. An imbalanced gut can lead to hormonal disruptions, affecting everything from sleep and mood to weight management and stress levels.
8. **Detoxification.** According to the National Institutes of Health, a healthy gut microbiome plays a crucial role in supporting liver function and aiding in detoxification. By helping the body process and eliminate toxins more efficiently, the gut reduces the risk of cellular damage and supports metabolic health.

9. **Mitochondrial health.** Mitochondria are the energy-producing structures within your cells—often referred to as the powerhouses of the cell. The metabolites produced by your gut bacteria can support mitochondrial function, which is essential for efficient energy production and overall cellular health. Maintaining healthy mitochondria is key to delaying the aging process and sustaining high energy levels throughout your life.
10. **Skin health.** The health of your gut directly affects the condition of your skin. A balanced microbiome can reduce skin inflammation and conditions like acne and eczema, leading to clearer, more youthful skin.

I truly believe that absolutely everyone should get a comprehensive stool analysis at least once in their lifetime to gain insights into their gut health. I'll discuss this more in the next chapter.

There's a reason your gut is called a "second brain," and my signature online program, GutBrain Method, helps my clients (and me) gain a new understanding of how food and high-quality supplement intake can help you heal the root cause of your issues and optimize your health with insights from the gut microbiome. Learn more at gutbrainmethod.com.

The Gut–Mental Health Connection

Your gut and brain are in constant communication via the gut-brain axis. What happens in your gut directly impacts your mood, focus, and overall mental health. As mentioned earlier, up to 90 percent of serotonin, the feel-good hormone that regulates emotional well-being, is produced in the gut, and your gut bacteria play a huge role in its production. If your gut is imbalanced, it's no wonder you might feel anxious or moody or have trouble concentrating.

As my colleague from Harvard, Dr. Uma Naidoo, often emphasizes, the gut-brain connection is a game-changer for mental health and emotional well-being. As a pioneer in the field of nutritional psychiatry, she has shown through her research how specific dietary interventions can help treat conditions like anxiety and depression. An imbalance in gut bacteria doesn't just affect digestion—it disrupts neurotransmitters like serotonin, dopamine, and gamma-aminobutyric acid (GABA), which regulate mood, motivation, and stress.

Nourishing your gut microbiome with the right foods is a positive step toward better mental health. These powerful tools support beneficial bacteria that influence neurotransmitter production. Prebiotic-rich foods also feed these good bacteria, helping to stabilize mood and reduce inflammation in the brain. In Chapter 5, I dive into the specific foods and strategies for improving your gut and brain health, guided by the science of nutritional psychiatry. For now, remember: Taking care of your gut means taking care of your mind!

Gut Health's Role in Food Sensitivities and Autoimmunity

A gut that isn't functioning properly can cause food allergies, intolerances, and sensitivities. Research indicates that conditions like celiac disease and nonceliac gluten sensitivity are directly linked to gut health. An unhealthy gut can also trigger autoimmune conditions by allowing undigested food particles and toxins to enter the bloodstream, leading to an immune response—so taking care of your gut is essential to keeping your body's defenses in check!

> If you want to improve serotonin production, stabilize your mood, and boost energy, what you eat matters.

Now let's get into the details.

Five Aspects of Optimal Gut Health

When we talk about optimal gut health, we're looking at five key factors that must be addressed: digestion, inflammation, microbiome and dysbiosis, detox and metabolic imbalances, and infections like parasites, fungi, or yeast. Each of these plays a vital role in how your body processes food, absorbs nutrients, and maintains a healthy metabolism. Let's start with digestion, the cornerstone of gut health.

1. Digestion and Absorption Essentials

Most people assume digestion occurs automatically. For the most part it does, but we can do things to make the process work better for our particular bodies. While the saying "You are what you eat" holds some truth, the real story lies in how effectively your body breaks down and absorbs what you consume. This complex process involves enzymes, bile, and a balanced microbiome working together to extract nutrients and eliminate waste.

For many over the age of forty, digestion doesn't work as smoothly as it once did. Stress, demanding schedules, and natural aging contribute to a decline in pancreatic function, making it harder to produce the enzymes needed to break down fats, proteins, and carbohydrates. This can lead to symptoms like bloating, constipation, and fatigue, and nutrient deficiencies can develop over time. Vitamins like A, D, E, and K—essential for healthy skin, energy, and immune function—may not be absorbed effectively.

A common but often overlooked issue is exocrine pancreatic insufficiency, where the pancreas struggles to produce enough digestive enzymes. This, combined with imbalances in the gut microbiome, can wreak havoc on digestion. One client, Gayle, age fifty-two, came to me with chronic bloating and constipation. Despite her healthy eating habits, she felt fatigued and depleted. After testing, I diagnosed her with enzymatic insufficiency and dysbiosis—a significant imbalance between beneficial and pathogenic bacteria in her gut.

We tackled Gayle's issues with a targeted plan:

- **Digestive enzymes.** I introduced a high-quality enzyme supplement to aid in breaking down fats and proteins.
- **Bitter greens and herbs.** She began incorporating bitter greens like dandelion and arugula into her meals, which naturally stimulate bile and enzyme production. I also recommended a few drops of Swedish bitters before meals to prepare her digestive system.
- **Restoring microbiome balance.** Gayle added probiotic-rich fermented foods and prebiotic vegetables like asparagus, and eliminated foods that encouraged bacterial overgrowth.
- **Breathwork before meals.** By taking three deep breaths before eating, Gayle activated her parasympathetic nervous system, calming her body and enhancing digestion.

Within weeks, Gayle's symptoms dramatically improved. She felt regular for the first time in years, her bloating disappeared, and her energy levels soared. She even noticed her skin and hair looking healthier, proof of the systemic benefits of proper digestion.

Pro Tip from a Dietitian

- For those looking to improve digestion and nutrient absorption, a multipronged approach can make all the difference. While I often prescribe digestive enzymes to support fat and protein breakdown, I also recommend incorporating bitter greens like arugula, dandelion, and radicchio into your meals. These greens naturally stimulate digestive enzymes and bile production, which are essential for breaking down fats and aiding overall digestion.
- For an extra boost, bitter herb tinctures such as Swedish bitters can be a game-changer. A few drops before meals help prime your digestive system, preparing it to process food efficiently. You can easily find them online or at most natural health stores. I go into more detail on their benefits a few pages ahead, so be sure to keep reading.
- The ultimate pro tip? **Breathwork.** Taking three deep breaths before eating shifts your body from a stressed, fight-or-flight state to a relaxed, rest-and-digest mode. This simple practice activates your parasympathetic nervous system, enhancing digestion and improving nutrient absorption. Combining these strategies can help you get the most out of every meal while reducing bloating and discomfort.

Optimal digestion isn't just about avoiding discomfort—it's about ensuring that your body gets the nutrients it needs to thrive. Small, intentional changes can transform your health, making every meal work for you.

Breathwork

Don't underestimate the power of breath. I've worked with many busy clients, including CEOs, and after guiding them through my nutrition program—eliminating artificial ingredients and improving their nutrient intake with high-quality supplements—they all found breathwork to be a key component of their transformation. They realized that taking a moment to pause and engage in breathwork before a meal not only helped them manage stress but also enhanced their enjoyment of food. Allowing yourself just ten minutes of stress-free, mindful eating can make your food taste even better.

A Three-Breath Practice to Activate Digestion

One of the simplest, most cost-effective ways to optimize digestion is to activate your parasympathetic nervous system—also known as the rest-and-digest state. This helps your body shift out of the sympathetic nervous system, which controls the fight-or-flight response during times of stress or intense focus.

Transitioning into a relaxed state before eating boosts the release of digestive enzymes and supports nutrient absorption. According to a 2020 study by Paul Lehrer published in *Neuroscience & Biobehavioral Reviews,* slow, controlled exhalation activates the vagus nerve, which signals safety to the brain and helps shift the body into a parasympathetic state, priming the digestive system to receive and process food efficiently.

Here's a three-breath practice you can use before meals:

- **First breath.** Pause for a moment, take a deep breath in, and gently exhale.
- **Second breath.** Inhale again, focusing on making the exhale longer than the inhale. This activates the vagus nerve.

- **Final breath.** With your third slow breath, you may notice your mouth begin to salivate—this is your gut-brain connection in action. That saliva isn't just moisture. It contains amylase, which begins the breakdown of carbohydrates, and lingual lipase, which initiates fat digestion. This mindful moment helps set the entire digestive process in motion—naturally, effectively, and scientifically.

Additionally, some people like to incorporate gratitude meditation before meals, as my role model Gisele Bündchen suggests. Taking a moment to say a prayer of thanks to everyone involved in bringing your meal to the table—from farmers and growers to pickers, delivery people, supermarket workers, and the person who cooked the meal—can be a powerful way to connect with your food and nourish yourself physically and emotionally.

Other Ways to Support Your Digestion

Disclaimer: Always consult with your healthcare provider before using any herbal treatments. This helps ensure that you create a personalized protocol that is safe and right for your unique needs.

Swedish bitters. Swedish bitters is a traditional herbal formula composed of various bitter herbs that stimulate digestive enzymes and bile production. Key ingredients include the following:

- **Gentian root.** Enhances gastric acid secretion and helps break down proteins.
- **Wormwood.** Promotes bile flow and supports healthy liver function.
- **Dandelion root.** Stimulates bile production and aids in detoxification.
- **Angelica root.** Improves digestive motility and helps alleviate bloating.

These herbs work synergistically to regulate stomach acidity, support liver function, and improve overall digestive efficiency. Taking Swedish bitters before or after meals can help relieve indigestion and enhance nutrient absorption.

Enzyme supplements. After doing a lot of gut health tests, I often find people dealing with enzyme deficiencies. Adding enzyme supplements can make a huge difference in how people feel—less constipation, less bloating, and just better overall digestion.

That said, not everyone needs to take digestive enzymes regularly—they're best used selectively, under guidance, especially if you have conditions like low stomach acid or pancreatic insufficiency, or experience persistent bloating or malabsorption. But if I was to generalize, I'd say people over forty with super-busy, high-stress lifestyles often benefit from a little extra digestive support.

Enzyme supplements help your body break down food more effectively, supporting nutrient absorption and reducing digestive discomfort. Some of my go-to enzymes are as follows. You can find high-quality versions at trusted health stores or through professional-grade platforms like Fullscript or Pure Encapsulations.

- **Pancreatic elastase.** A crucial enzyme produced by the pancreas that helps break down proteins into smaller peptides so that your body can absorb them better, supporting protein digestion and absorption.
- **Lipase.** Breaks fats down into fatty acids and glycerol, making them easier to digest.
- **Amylase.** Breaks carbs down into simple sugars, which your body can absorb more easily.
- **Protease.** Helps digest proteins into amino acids, which are super important for muscle repair and overall health.

Taking enzyme supplements with each meal can significantly improve digestion, reduce bloating, and enhance nutrient uptake, especially for those with pancreatic insufficiency or suboptimal enzyme production. If you're feeling bloated or sluggish after meals, adding the right enzyme might be just what you need.

2. Inflammation of the Gut Lining: Understanding Leaky Gut

Inflammation of the gut lining—leaky gut—is one of the most critical factors affecting gut health. The gut lining acts as a barrier, protecting your body from harmful substances like toxins, undigested food particles, and pathogens. When this protective layer becomes compromised—due to stress, microbial imbalances, or inflammatory foods—microscopic gaps form, allowing these harmful substances to pass into the bloodstream. This process triggers systemic inflammation, which can manifest as fatigue, joint pain, skin issues, food sensitivities, and even autoimmune conditions.

One of my clients, Sophia, age forty-seven, experienced this firsthand. Despite eating what she thought was a healthy diet, she struggled with autoimmune conditions and felt fatigued and plagued by joint discomfort. Testing revealed elevated levels of calprotectin, a marker of intestinal inflammation, and low secretory immunoglobulin A (IgA), an essential antibody for gut immune defense. These findings confirmed the presence of leaky gut. We took a focused approach to address the root cause of her inflammation:

- **Gut barrier repair.** Sophia began supplementing with SBI Protect (immunoglobulin colostrum and serum-derived bovine immunoglobulin) to strengthen the gut lining.
- **Inflammation reduction.** She transitioned to an anti-inflammatory protocol to calm her gut, detailed in Chapter 5,

which includes dietary adjustments and key anti-inflammatory nutrients.

- **Microbial balance.** We introduced specific probiotics and prebiotics to restore her gut microbiome, helping crowd out harmful bacteria and promote healing.

Within weeks, Sophia's symptoms improved significantly. Her joint pain eased, her energy returned, and she no longer felt bloated after meals. This transformation highlights how reducing gut inflammation can ripple out to positively impact the entire body.

Stress and Gut Inflammation

Chronic stress plays a major role in gut inflammation by increasing cortisol levels. Elevated cortisol weakens the tight junctions in the gut lining, making it more permeable and prone to inflammation. Stress also suppresses secretory IgA, reducing the gut's ability to fight off harmful pathogens. This combination creates a perfect storm for leaky gut to develop and worsen. In Sophia's case, stress was a major contributor to her symptoms. By incorporating simple breathwork techniques, mindfulness practices, and gentle movement, we reduced her cortisol levels, which supported her gut's healing process.

Testing for Inflammation

Comprehensive gut health testing provides key insights into inflammation and its underlying causes. Biomarkers like these can reveal the state of your gut health:

- **Calprotectin.** Detects intestinal inflammation, often linked to inflammatory bowel diseases.
- **Secretory IgA.** Reflects immune defense in the gut; low levels indicate stress or weakened immunity.

- **Eosinophil Protein X.** Measures allergic or inflammatory activity in the gut lining.

These tests are typically not covered by insurance as they fall under the category of advanced or functional diagnostics. However, many clients find them worthwhile for personalized care. Out-of-pocket costs generally range from $300 to $500, depending on the lab and depth of analysis.

The Role of Food in Gut Inflammation

While stress and microbial imbalances are significant factors, inflammatory foods like refined sugars, gluten, and processed oils can further damage the gut lining. The next chapter provides a complete guide to identifying and eliminating inflammatory foods while incorporating anti-inflammatory ones to support gut healing. Remember: *What you eat affects how you think and feel.* Chronic inflammation in the gut, often caused by a poor diet, damages the gut lining and disrupts this connection, leading to mental health issues like anxiety and depression. By focusing on gut-friendly, nutrient-dense foods, you can strengthen the gut-brain axis and transform your mental clarity and emotional resilience.

Pro Tip from a Dietitian

To address gut inflammation,

- Repair the gut lining with supplements like immunoglobulin colostrum and SBI Protect.
- Manage stress with daily breathwork or mindfulness to lower cortisol and improve gut barrier function.
- Reduce dietary inflammation by following an anti-inflammatory diet. For specific food recommendations, see Chapter 5.

Addressing inflammation at the gut level is transformative, resolving not just digestive discomfort but also systemic issues like fatigue, joint pain, and immune dysfunction. The gut truly is the gateway to overall health, and controlling inflammation is the key to unlocking its potential.

3. Microbiome: Supporting Healthy Diversity

Your GI microbiome is like a bustling city, home to trillions of bacteria that play critical roles in digestion, immunity, mood, and energy levels. Maintaining diversity in this ecosystem is essential for gut health, and the key lies both in what you eat and how you support your microbiome.

One client, Daniel, age forty-two, came to me feeling constantly fatigued, frequently sick, and struggling to lose weight despite eating a clean diet of simple, whole foods without artificial ingredients. Testing revealed a lack of microbial diversity, including low levels of *Akkermansia muciniphila*, a bacterium crucial for maintaining gut barrier integrity and regulating metabolism. With a few targeted changes—incorporating prebiotics, polyphenol-rich foods, and rotating probiotics—Daniel saw dramatic improvements in energy, fewer illnesses, and better metabolic health within a few months.

To support a thriving microbiome, it's important to combine probiotics and prebiotics strategically. **Probiotics** are the live bacteria found in fermented foods like yogurt, kefir, and kimchi or in supplements, and they directly replenish beneficial strains in your gut. **Prebiotics**, on the other hand, are nondigestible fibers that feed these bacteria, helping them grow and thrive. Foods like garlic, onions, green bananas, and cooked-and-cooled potatoes are excellent sources of prebiotics. When it comes to potatoes, all varieties can offer this benefit, but they must be fully cooled after cooking to form resistant starch, the type of prebiotic that supports gut health. While cold is ideal, room temperature is generally sufficient to preserve the resistant starch content.

For those with specific microbial imbalances, like low levels of *Akkermansia,* certain polyphenol-rich foods can be particularly helpful. Research shows that polyphenol-rich foods such as cranberries, pomegranates, and green tea encourage the growth of this critical bacterium, which supports gut-lining integrity and reduces inflammation.

Diverse prebiotic fibers are crucial for feeding a range of beneficial bacteria. For example,

- **Inulin,** found in chicory root, garlic, and onions, supports bacteria like *Akkermansia.*
- **Resistant starch,** present in green bananas and cooked and cooled potatoes, fuels bacteria that produce short-chain fatty acids to reduce inflammation.
- **Fructooligosaccharides (FOS)** in asparagus and bananas feed bacteria like *Lactobacillus* and *Bifidobacterium*, essential for gut balance.

To maximize diversity, don't just stick to one type of fiber or bacteria—variety is key. Each type of food and probiotic strain supports different functions, contributing to a balanced, resilient microbiome.

Pro Tip from a Dietitian

Here's the secret sauce to gut health: Rotate your probiotics every ninety days and eat thirty or more different vegetables each week. This number comes from the **American Gut Project,** one of the largest microbiome studies to date, which found that people who ate **thirty or more types of plant foods per week** had significantly more diverse gut microbiomes than those who ate fewer than ten—an important marker of better digestive, immune, and metabolic health. I know that may sound like a lot—especially when most people struggle to meet even the basic fruit and vegetable recommendations—but the key is **variety over volume.** Think small servings, creative combinations, and building diversity over time, not perfection in a single week. Switching probiotics ensures that your microbiome gets exposed to a variety of strains, which strengthens gut diversity. For example, start with a *Lactobacillus-Bifidobacterium* blend, then move to one that includes *Akkermansia*-supportive strains.

On the food side, aim for variety in your produce aisle. Try that kohlrabi you've never cooked before, add bok choy to stir-fries, or throw radishes into your salads. Research shows that eating a diverse range of plant-based foods supports a healthier microbiome, boosting immunity, improving digestion, and even regulating your mood.

Your gut thrives on diversity. Treat it like a dynamic ecosystem—mix things up, try new foods, and rotate your probiotics. It's not just about gut health; it's about creating a foundation for energy, resilience, and well-being.

4. Gut Microbiome Metabolites: The Role of SCFAs and Beta-Glucuronidase

Not many people realize that our gut's function goes far beyond digestion and nutrient absorption. It also plays a vital role in metabolizing compounds that influence everything from immunity to hormone balance. Key players in this process include short-chain fatty acids (SCFAs) and beta-glucuronidase, metabolites that are produced or influenced by your gut microbiome.

SCFAs—like acetate, propionate, and butyrate—are produced when gut bacteria ferment dietary fibers and resistant starches. These metabolites are crucial for maintaining health. They have anti-inflammatory and immunoregulatory effects, helping to reduce inflammation and modulate immune responses to protect against chronic diseases. SCFAs also support metabolic health by improving insulin sensitivity, aiding in weight management, and lowering the risk of type 2 diabetes. Additionally, butyrate fuels colon cells, maintains gut lining integrity, and supports brain health by reducing neuroinflammation.

As a dietitian, I use comprehensive gut health testing as part of my Gut-Brain Method to assess how well my clients' microbiomes produce SCFAs and support detoxification pathways. This test provides insights into how effectively their gut microbiome is working and helps identify areas for improvement.

The best way to increase SCFA levels is by embracing a fiber-rich, plant-forward diet such as the Mediterranean diet. This diet emphasizes a variety of fruits, vegetables, whole grains, and legumes—all of which provide the fermentable fibers that bacteria use to produce SCFAs. Including prebiotic foods like garlic, onions, asparagus, and artichokes in your meals can further enhance SCFA production. Resistant starches from cooked and cooled potatoes, green bananas, and legumes are another excellent way to fuel SCFA-producing bacteria. For individuals with particularly low SCFA levels, butyrate supplementation can provide targeted support, especially for gut-lining integrity and inflammation control.

Vitamin K

Another critical metabolite produced by the gut microbiome is vitamin K, a nutrient essential for blood clotting and bone health. The microbiome synthesizes vitamin K during fermentation, so including fermented foods like sauerkraut, kimchi, and miso can naturally support your levels. Eating a diverse, plant-rich diet also ensures that your gut bacteria have the resources to produce this important vitamin.

Dangers of Too Much Red Meat and Elevated Metabolites

While many metabolites are beneficial, some, like beta-glucuronidase, can cause problems when elevated. High levels of this enzyme can interfere with estrogen metabolism, leading to hormone imbalances. To lower beta-glucuronidase levels, it's important to limit red meat intake to no more than one to two times per week and no more than four to five times per month to balance nutrient intake. Adding glucuronic acid–rich foods like apples, citrus fruits, and broccoli can also help neutralize the effects of elevated beta-glucuronidase. Konjac root, a plant native to Asia, is rich in glucomannan, a type of soluble fiber that supports gut health, blood sugar balance, and gentle detoxification. It's commonly found in supplement form and also made into low-carb, high-fiber noodles—often called shirataki noodles. Both forms can be beneficial, though the supplement typically delivers a more concentrated dose of fiber, which is another effective addition to support gut health and detoxification.

Pro Tip from a Dietitian

Focus on a diverse, fiber-rich diet that includes prebiotic and fermented foods. Try rotating new vegetables into your meals each week, such as artichokes, green bananas, or konjac root, to feed a broader range of beneficial bacteria. These small but intentional changes will empower your microbiome to produce the metabolites your body needs to thrive.

5. Gut Infections: Parasites and Yeast (Candida)

Now that we have covered digestion, nutrient absorption, and the microbiome, it is crucial to understand and address infections from yeast, fungi, viruses, and parasites. These unwanted intruders can disrupt the delicate balance of your gut microbiome, leading to a wide range of symptoms that affect not only digestion but also skin, mood, energy levels, and even immunity.

Keep in mind that maintaining a healthy gut microbiome strengthens your immune system, which in turn prevents opportunistic infections. As we've discussed, up to 80 percent of your immune system is housed in the gut—specifically, the gut-associated lymphoid tissue (GALT), where the microbiome plays a critical role in modulating immune responses and preventing overgrowth of harmful pathogens. When you take care of one aspect, it automatically supports the others.

Why is this important? Gut infections often go undetected, yet they are the root cause of many chronic issues. Parasites can cause nutrient malabsorption and systemic symptoms like fatigue and muscle pain while yeast overgrowth, like candida, thrives in an imbalanced gut, leading to bloating, brain fog, and skin conditions. Identifying and treating these infections is essential to restoring balance and optimizing your gut health.

Parasitic Infections

Parasitic infections can present with a wide range of symptoms, depending on the type of organism, its location in the body, and the severity of the infection. Common signs include digestive issues like bloating, diarrhea, abdominal pain, and constipation, as well as systemic symptoms such as fatigue, muscle aches, brain fog, or skin irritation.

While some parasites—such as giardia and *Entamoeba histolytica* —are more common in developing countries due to contaminated water or poor sanitation, others are surprisingly common in everyday life. For example, anisakis, a parasite found in raw or undercooked fish (like sushi), can cause symptoms that mimic food poisoning, including nausea, vomiting, and abdominal pain shortly after eating.

Because parasitic infections often go undiagnosed, I recommend comprehensive stool testing for clients with persistent or unexplained symptoms—especially if they've traveled internationally or frequently consume raw fish or unwashed produce.

Once identified, parasites can be addressed with natural antimicrobials such as black walnut hull, wormwood, oregano oil, clove oil, and grapefruit seed extract—all of which have strong antiparasitic properties while also supporting microbial balance and gut lining repair.

How I Diagnosed Myself with Parasites

Even as a gut health expert, I'm not impervious or immune to the unexpected. A couple of years ago, I developed an eczema-like rash on my wrist and the following month on my chest, along with bloating and low energy. After topical treatments failed, I suspected the root cause to be in my gut. A comprehensive stool test confirmed I had dysbiosis and a parasitic infection.

The connection between my gut and skin was clear: The imbalance in my microbiome was impacting my digestion, mood, and overall health. I developed a treatment protocol for myself that included *Saccharomyces boulardii* probiotics; herbal antimicrobials like clove, thyme, and oregano oil; and an intermittent fasting protocol with a sixteen-hour fasting window. Within a month, the eczema disappeared, my energy improved, and my skin issues have not returned!

Action Steps for Parasites

1. **Test.** Consult your healthcare provider and get a stool test to confirm parasitic infections.
2. **Treat.** Use herbal antimicrobials like black walnut (250 mg three times daily), wormwood (200 mg three times daily), and oregano oil (500 mg four times daily). For more serious or confirmed parasitic infections, a healthcare provider may prescribe **antiparasitic or antibiotic medications,** such as

metronidazole or albendazole, depending on the organism. In such cases, **natural antimicrobials** like black walnut, wormwood, or oregano oil may still be used, but they should be taken under professional guidance.

3. **Support healing.** Include activated charcoal during treatment to bind and eliminate toxins and follow up with probiotics to rebalance your microbiome.

Candida Overgrowth

Candida yeast naturally exists in small amounts in the gut, skin, and mucous membranes. However, when the balance of the gut microbiome is disrupted by factors like antibiotic use, high-sugar diets, or chronic stress, candida can overgrow, leading to symptoms like bloating, brain fog, fatigue, white coating on the tongue, vaginal discharge, and skin rashes.

How Candida Overgrowth Happens

- **Antibiotic use.** Wipes out beneficial bacteria, allowing candida to grow unchecked.
- **High-sugar diets.** Constant snacking and drinking sugary beverages fuel candida overgrowth as it thrives on sugar and refined carbs.
- **Weakened immune system.** Chronic stress, lack of sleep, and illness reduce the body's defenses.
- **Hormonal imbalances.** Chronically elevated insulin from high carbohydrate intake, birth control pills, or menopause-related changes can encourage candida growth.

Left untreated, candida overgrowth disrupts the gut-brain axis, contributing to inflammation, poor nutrient absorption, vaginal yeast infection, and weakened immunity.

Action Steps for Candida

1. **Diet.** Eliminate sugar and processed carbs. Focus on alkalizing foods like kale, spinach, broccoli, and bitter greens such as arugula and radicchio.
2. **Antifungal foods.** Incorporate garlic, oregano oil, and caprylic acid for their natural antifungal properties.
3. **Supplements.** Undecylenic acid is highly effective for inhibiting candida and balancing gut flora. Pair with probiotics containing *Lactobacillus* and *Bifidobacterium* strains.
4. **Lifestyle.** Reduce stress and ensure adequate sleep to strengthen immunity and support microbiome balance.

Pro Tip from a Dietitian

If you suspect gut infections like parasites or candida, always start with a stool test. It's the most reliable way to identify the problem. For parasites, use a combination of herbal antimicrobials and support detox with activated charcoal. For candida, cutting out sugar is essential, and adding bitter greens, antifungal foods, and probiotics can help restore balance.

Your gut health plays a central role in digestion, immunity, and skin health. By addressing infections and rebalancing your microbiome, you can resolve stubborn symptoms and improve your overall well-being. In the next two chapters, I share the top foods and lifestyle tips for healing your gut for better health and vitality.

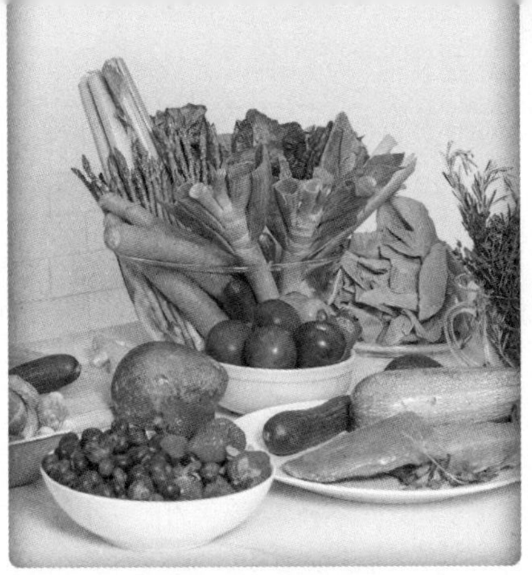

Chapter 3
Get to Know Your Bio-Individuality: Seven Tools to Consider

HAVE YOU EVER WONDERED why we *still* don't have a definitive answer to this seemingly simple question: *What is the best diet for humans?*

The concept of dieting has been around for well over a century. The first widely recognized diet book was published in 1863 by William Banting, titled *Letter on Corpulence, Addressed to the Public.* It promoted a low-carbohydrate, high-protein diet, which shares similarities with modern ketogenic diets.

Later, in 1918, Lulu Hunt Peters introduced the idea of calorie counting in her book *Diet & Health: With Key to the Calories.* This book popularized the concept of managing weight through caloric restriction and became a bestseller, significantly influencing the dieting culture we know today.

These early works laid the foundation for the many diet debates and methodologies we now see. However, after more than a century of research and experimentation, we still don't have a universal answer to what constitutes the best diet for everyone, largely because human health is highly individual, and nutrient needs differ greatly from person to person.

Perhaps the reason we still don't have the answer is that *we've been asking ourselves the wrong question.*

Maybe we've been asking the wrong question because the answer really lies within the human body itself. Could the answer be in your health conditions, your DNA, your age, your gender, your body's metabolism, your hormones, and your unique bio-individuality?

Which Diet Is Best for Humans?

As a dietitian, I see so much confusion about whether a vegan, plant-based diet or a carnivorous, high-protein diet is healthier. "Should I be vegan or paleo? A vegetarian or a pescetarian?" are questions I'm asked all the time. The answer, for most people, is neither. What you really need is to get to know your own body to find what's right for you—and become a you-tarian who simply eats what your body loves!

I have clients who have come to me because they're "doing keto," but they're not really in ketosis. It makes them feel good to say that they're doing keto because at one point this was the cool diet for overachievers and hardcore folks. They may have lost a little weight from giving up refined, processed carbs (which is a good thing), but now their digestion is a mess from eating heavy cream and processed, prepackaged keto-branded meals and desserts. They're not paying attention to how they're feeling and the messages their body is sending about how these foods impact them.

On the other end of the spectrum, I have worked with many women who are proud vegans living a plant-based lifestyle. They are passionate about their food philosophy and often worry that they're "not plant-based enough" or "not raw enough," so they keep pushing harder toward a diet made up of veggies, fruits, nuts, and grains. But then they're confused because they're still struggling with poor digestion, autoimmune diseases, and most of all, hormonal imbalances. Their bodies need good-quality protein and healthy fats to stay in balance, particularly at certain times during their cycle (more on that later). They're not listening to the symptoms that are telling them that their diet isn't working for them.

In reality, many individual factors—including genetics, lifestyle, hormonal makeup, and microbial composition—determine whether a plant-based diet or one that's higher in animal fats is best for us.

In this chapter, we build on the basics of gut health by learning how *you specifically* should be eating based on your own bio-individuality. This is about getting to know—and love—your own body. I want you to become enchanted with your gut, your blood sugar, your hormones, and lymphatic system. Because when you really love something, you take care of it. You pay attention. You take the time to figure out what it needs, what works and doesn't work. This is different for everyone, which is why diet trends and food fads can be so confusing. While general principles of nutrition apply in most cases, ultimately no meal is universally accepted as neutral or healthy for everyone, regardless of individual differences—no "Switzerland meal."

On the following pages, I walk you step-by-step through the process of developing a personalized nutrition plan based on your bio-individuality—the unique physiological and lifestyle factors that make you *you*, including your genetics, lifestyle, stress levels, metabolism, hormonal makeup, and activity levels. Together, these factors determine how your body responds to different foods. More and more research is showing that a personalized approach to nutrition based on bio-individuality is more effective than any one diet approach—including the Mediterranean diet, which is generally considered the gold standard for disease prevention, weight loss, and longevity.

I'll help you gather critical data points from your own body, including:

- *Your genetics and ancestry*, which determine what kind of diet (more plant-based or higher in animal protein and healthy fats) your body is optimized to thrive on
- *Your level of glucose sensitivity*, which can help you determine how your body responds to sugar and carbohydrates (If you're of European or Jewish descent, you might be more sensitive than you realize!)
- For women, *your hormonal makeup*, which means that you thrive on different foods every week of the month
- *Food sensitivities, intolerances, and allergies* that may be undermining your health without your awareness

By going through my list of seven big questions to unlock your bio-individuality—including DIY approaches and professional testing options to help you find answers—you'll have everything you need to design your own you-tarian diet.

As a longevity and gut health dietitian, I believe that understanding your unique bio-individuality is the key to optimizing your health and extending your lifespan. We all have distinct needs, and what works for one person may not work for another. For example, if you're of northern European or Ashkenazi Jewish descent, your genetic background may increase your risk for certain gut-related or autoimmune conditions, making it especially important to understand your bio-individual needs. Or if you're a woman, your hormonal fluctuations mean you may need different foods each week of the month—to support shifting levels of estrogen, progesterone, and insulin sensitivity, and to help stabilize energy, mood, and digestion throughout your cycle.

That's where advanced testing comes into play. By using these cutting-edge tools, you can gain deep insights into how your body functions and tailor your diet, lifestyle, and supplements for optimal health.

Here are the top seven tools I recommend for understanding your unique bio-individuality and improving your health journey:

- DNA methylation (epigenetic age) testing
- Comprehensive gut microbiome testing
- Advanced nutrient testing for 242 biomarkers
- Fasting insulin testing
- Continuous glucose monitoring
- Determining food sensitivities and intolerances
- Hormonal testing

1. DNA Testing and the Power of Personalized Health

Understanding your body's unique genetic and biological blueprint is a game-changer when it comes to optimizing health. DNA testing, particularly DNA methylation tests, provides critical insights into how your genes are expressed and how your lifestyle choices impact your biological age. Unlike your chronological age, which simply counts the years you've lived, your biological age reflects the condition of your cells and their rate of aging.

One of the most advanced tools I use with my clients is the DNA methylation test, specifically the TruDiagnostic test. This test measures DNA methylation patterns, which are chemical changes that regulate gene expression. These patterns are influenced by your environment, diet, and habits, making them a dynamic marker of your health. The results reveal your biological age and provide a clear picture of how well your body is aging at the cellular level.

Take Sarah, age fifty, for example. Although she appeared to be in good physical shape—exercising a few times a week and maintaining a healthy weight—her DNA methylation test revealed her biological age was fifty-eight, a full eight years older than her chronological age.

Digging deeper, we discovered she was eating a highly inflammatory diet—heavy in processed snacks, low in fiber and antioxidants—and often skipped meals due to a demanding work schedule. She averaged only five to six hours of sleep per night, regularly worked late, and felt constantly wired but exhausted. While she exercised occasionally, it was inconsistent and lacked restorative movement like stretching or mindfulness-based activity.

We created a personalized plan that addressed these root causes: introducing methylation-supportive nutrients such as folate, B_6, and B_{12}; reducing processed and inflammatory foods; improving sleep hygiene; and incorporating daily stress-reducing practices like yoga and breathwork.

Within a year, Sarah's biological age decreased by five years—and more importantly, she reported feeling clearer, calmer, and more energized than she had in over a decade.

Methylation plays a critical role in processes essential to your overall health, including detoxification, hormone regulation, cardiovascular function, and cellular energy production. Take Mark, age thirty-nine, for example. A busy tech executive and new father, he often skipped meals, relied heavily on caffeine, and got by on just five to six hours of sleep per night. Despite regular workouts, he struggled with chronic brain fog, low motivation, and afternoon crashes that left him feeling frustrated and disconnected. Genetic testing revealed a methylation inefficiency (specifically MTHFR and COMT variants) that impacted his neurotransmitter production, including dopamine and serotonin—key regulators of mood, energy, and focus. This discovery finally explained the symptoms he had long dismissed as "just stress."

We designed a targeted protocol that prioritized choline-rich foods like eggs and grass-fed beef liver, added magnesium glycinate, and included methylated B vitamins (B_6, B_{12}, and folate) to support his unique genetic profile. Within six weeks, Mark reported sharper focus, a more stable mood, and fewer energy crashes—feeling more like himself than he had in years. Why does this matter? Because understanding your biological age and methylation efficiency gives you the power to make data-driven decisions that directly influence your longevity. By identifying inefficiencies, you can adopt targeted interventions to slow cellular aging, improve energy, and enhance overall health.

DNA testing isn't just about solving problems—it's about maximizing potential. It helps you understand how your genetics influence nutrient absorption, detoxification, and even your risk for certain conditions. This knowledge enables you to create a diet and lifestyle that align with your unique biology, ensuring that every choice you make supports your health and longevity. When you know better, you can do better—and the results can be life-changing.

2. Comprehensive Gut Health Test: The Key to Optimal Health

Next is my favorite test, the one that changed my life and helps my clients understand the root cause of mini-imbalances. You learned about the second brain in Chapter 2. The comprehensive gut test provides an in-depth look at what's happening inside your digestive system, offering insights into the health of your microbiome and its impact on everything from digestion to mental clarity.

This test evaluates key markers such as maldigestion, inflammation, dysbiosis, metabolite imbalances, and infections like parasites or yeast overgrowth. These factors can disrupt your gut's ability to function optimally, affecting not just digestion but also your energy levels, metabolism, and immune system.

One of my clients, Lisa, age thirty-six, came to me with persistent bloating, fatigue, and skin issues, including adult acne along her jawline and recurring eczema flare-ups. She had tried multiple topical treatments with little success, not realizing the root cause was likely internal—in her gut. Her gut microbiome test revealed significant dysbiosis, with low levels of beneficial bacteria, overgrowth of yeast, and pancreatic enzyme insufficiency. By incorporating enzymes, probiotics tailored to her needs, prebiotic-rich foods like asparagus and onions, and a temporary elimination of sugar to starve yeast overgrowth, Lisa saw great improvements. Within weeks, her bloating was gone, her energy was back, and her skin cleared up!

The gut microbiome also plays a critical role in mental health, as it directly influences neurotransmitter production. Another client, Tom, age forty-two, struggled with low energy, brain fog, and frequent digestive discomfort, including bloating and irregular bowel movements, which his test revealed were linked to high levels of inflammation in his gut and an overgrowth of pathogenic bacteria. With a protocol that included anti-inflammatory foods like turmeric and omega-3s, as well as gut-healing supplements like glutamine and mucosal lining repair supplements, Tom experienced better mental clarity and significant stamina improvements.

Why does this test matter? Optimal gut health enhances optimal nutrient digestion, boosts immunity, reduces inflammation, and even improves energy and mental clarity. *Testing your gut health allows you to address the root cause of symptoms rather than just managing them.* By identifying imbalances in your gut microbiome, you can take targeted steps to optimize nutrient absorption, support your immune system, and create a foundation for long-term health. If you've ever felt that something is off, this test can provide the answers you need to restore balance and thrive. (For more on gut health, refer back to Chapter 2.)

3. Advanced Nutrient Testing: Pinpointing Hidden Deficiencies and Toxins

When was the last time you felt truly energized, sharp, and balanced? For many, the answer is "Too long ago" or "I don't remember." Nutritional deficiencies and toxicities often go unnoticed until they manifest as persistent fatigue, weakened immunity, hormonal imbalances, or even mental fog and mood swings. Advanced nutrient testing for 242 biomarkers is a powerful tool that provides a detailed snapshot of your body's internal nutrient landscape, uncovering the root causes of these symptoms. This comprehensive test measures critical markers, such as

- **Hormones.** Balancing cortisol, thyroid, and reproductive hormones
- **Vitamins and minerals.** Detecting deficiencies in key nutrients like vitamin D and B_{12}, magnesium, and zinc
- **Iron levels.** Evaluating ferritin and iron-binding capacity to address anemia or overload
- **Organic acids.** Pinpointing metabolic inefficiencies that affect energy production and detoxification
- **Toxic metals.** Identifying harmful levels of lead, mercury, or arsenic that can sabotage your cellular health
- **Liver function.** Monitoring enzymes to assess detoxification capacity and overall liver health

Take Martha, age forty-eight, who came to me with chronic fatigue and difficulty losing weight. Despite eating a "clean high-protein diet," her nutrient test revealed critically low vitamin D and magnesium levels, combined with elevated levels of toxic aluminum. By supplementing with magnesium glycinate, increasing her vitamin D levels through cod liver oil and safe sun exposure, and replacing aluminum-containing products—such as cookware and canned foods—with stainless steel and ceramic alternatives and fresh, whole foods, Martha regained her energy and experienced noticeable improvements in both her vitality and lean body mass within weeks.

Another client, James, age thirty-four, was struggling with persistent anxiety, rapid weight loss, digestive discomfort, and difficulty concentrating—symptoms that began affecting his performance at work and his overall quality of life. His test showed low alpha-lipoic acid (ALA) levels and deficiencies in B vitamins essential for energy production. We added organ meats, leafy greens, and a high-quality methylated B-complex supplement to his routine. Within a month, James reported better metabolism and more stable moods, allowing him to excel in his demanding schedule as a financial analyst, where focus and high performance are critical.

Optimizing your nutrient levels is like fine-tuning a high-performance engine. Your body works better when every system is running at its best. Adequate levels of vitamins, minerals, and antioxidants are essential for

- **Energy production:** ensuring your mitochondria have the tools to generate sustained energy
- **Immune resilience:** fortifying your defenses against chronic infections and inflammation
- **Hormonal balance:** stabilizing cortisol, estrogen, and testosterone for better mood, metabolism, and vitality
- **Cellular detoxification:** removing harmful toxins that disrupt your metabolism and cause premature aging

Pro Tip from a Dietitian:

- If your test reveals deficiencies, start with food first. For example, organ meats like liver are nutrient powerhouses rich in iron, vitamin A, and alpha-lipoic acid.
- For toxic metal detoxification, focus on chelating foods like cilantro and chlorella, and work with a qualified practitioner for structured support—such as the "Push-Catch" method developed by Dr. Christopher Shade,

founder of Quicksilver Scientific. Dr. Shade offers extensive training for practitioners, and his protocols are used in integrative medicine. More information is available at quicksilverscientific.com.

- Use supplements strategically—choose forms your body can absorb, like magnesium glycinate, methylated B vitamins, or liposomal vitamin C. While some of these are available at health stores, higher-quality, practitioner-grade versions are typically found online or through specialty health retailers.

Symptoms like exhaustion, frequent colds, or difficulty concentrating aren't normal—they're your body's way of signaling that something is missing. Advanced nutrient testing gives you the data to fix what's broken and the confidence to take control of your health. With precise insights, you can rebuild your energy, sharpen your mind, and balance your body, ensuring you thrive—not just survive.

4. Fasting Insulin Test: The Key to Unlocking Metabolic Health

Remember how I said that your metabolism doesn't have to slow down when you age? Insulin resistance often operates in the shadows, quietly paving the way for weight gain, fatigue, and even diabetes long before these symptoms become obvious. But here is how to ensure a healthy metabolism: The fasting insulin test is a powerful diagnostic tool that reveals how efficiently your body processes glucose and how sensitive it is to insulin. High fasting insulin levels are an early warning sign that your body is struggling, providing a crucial opportunity to make changes before metabolic issues escalate.

When Melissa, age forty-two, first came to me, she was frustrated by stubborn weight gain despite exercising regularly and eating what she considered a healthy diet. She felt constantly tired, particularly in the afternoons, and struggled with sugar cravings that felt impossible to ignore. Her fasting insulin test revealed that her fasting insulin levels were significantly elevated, even though her blood glucose levels were still within the normal range. This was a clear indication of early-stage insulin resistance—a condition that, left unaddressed, could have progressed to diabetes. Armed with this knowledge, we implemented a targeted plan:

- **Diet adjustments.** Melissa shifted to a low-glycemic diet, focusing on whole, unprocessed foods like proteins at every meal, nonstarchy green and colorful vegetables, and healthy fats. She also replaced carbohydrates with fiber-rich alternatives like quinoa, beans, and lentils.
- **Time-restricted eating.** She adopted a 12:12 fasting schedule, giving her body time to stabilize insulin levels overnight and avoiding food intake at least three to four hours before bedtime.
- **Strength training.** Adding two thirty-minute strength-training sessions per week helped her build muscle, a key factor in improving insulin sensitivity.

Within three months, Melissa's insulin levels dropped by 25 percent, her energy returned, and she began losing weight effortlessly—without ever feeling deprived. More importantly, her risk of diabetes was significantly reduced, and she felt empowered to maintain these changes for life. High fasting insulin levels can remain hidden for years while quietly wreaking havoc on your metabolism. This condition is typically identified through a fasting insulin blood test, which is different from a standard fasting glucose test and provides earlier insight into insulin resistance—often before blood sugar levels begin to rise. Addressing insulin resistance early helps to prevent type 2 diabetes and supports weight loss because insulin sensitivity improves your ability to burn fat instead of storing it, to boost energy levels, and to increase the chances of health span for longevity. Lower insulin levels reduce inflammation and metabolic stress, key factors in healthy aging.

The fasting insulin test is more than just a number—it's often a wake-up call for men and women, typically around the age of forty to forty-five, when early signs of metabolic slowdown and insulin resistance can begin to surface. Whether you're battling chronic fatigue or working toward better metabolic health, this test provides the clarity you need to take control of your future. It's not about restriction—it's about understanding what your body needs to thrive and making choices that truly work for you!

I fell in love with taking care of my insulin for a deeply personal reason—my grandmother passed away at just sixty-two years old due to complications from diabetes. Knowing that I'm genetically predisposed to losing insulin sensitivity has driven me to take proactive steps to safeguard my health. Research shows that insulin resistance is a precursor to many chronic conditions, including type 2 diabetes, cardiovascular disease, and even cognitive decline. Studies have also demonstrated that maintaining hemoglobin A1c levels below 5.4 percent significantly reduces the risk of developing diabetes and related complications.

That's why I've mastered the low-carbohydrate diet and learned to genuinely enjoy it. A low-carb diet is scientifically proven to stabilize blood sugar, lower fasting insulin levels, and improve overall metabolic health. My home is 100 percent sugar-free, and I make it a priority to follow a low-carb diet at least 80 percent of the time—including limiting high-sugar foods and alcohol, which can quietly spike blood sugar and disrupt metabolic balance. This practice has helped me keep my hemoglobin A1c in the optimal range and maintain insulin sensitivity. I can't stress enough how important it is for everyone to start paying attention to these markers. It's one of the most effective ways to take control of your health and longevity.

5. Continuous Glucose Monitoring: A Window into Your Metabolism

One of the most powerful tools I use to help clients understand how food impacts their metabolism is a continuous glucose monitor (CGM). Unlike traditional blood sugar tests that provide a one-time snapshot, a CGM tracks your glucose levels in real time, 24/7, for up to fourteen days. This gives you a complete picture of how your body responds to everything—meals, workouts, stress, sleep, and even that post-dinner dessert.

Why does this matter? Because glucose spikes and crashes are the root cause of many energy dips, cravings, mood swings, and even long-term health issues like insulin resistance. By tracking your blood sugar in real time, you can see how your body reacts to specific foods and learn to make smarter, more informed choices.

One client, Anna, age thirty-four, loved starting her mornings with a smoothie packed with fruit, oats, and almond milk. Her CGM revealed a huge glucose spike right after breakfast, followed by an energy crash midmorning that left her reaching for coffee and snacks. By tweaking her smoothie—adding protein powder and healthy fats like almond butter and reducing the amount of fruit—her glucose curve flattened, and she noticed a major boost in energy and focus throughout the day. This is where tips from biochemist Jessie Inchauspé, a colleague of mine who made her entire career around CGM insights and is known as "Glucose Goddess," come in handy. For example,

- **Eat food in the right order.** Start with fiber and greens, followed by protein and fats, and save carbs for last. This simple shift can reduce glucose spikes by up to 30 percent.
- **Pair your carbs wisely.** If you love bread, add a spread of avocado or pair it with eggs. Fats and proteins slow down the absorption of glucose, leading to a more stable blood sugar response.
- **Use movement strategically.** A quick ten-minute walk after a meal can cut a glucose spike in half, helping your body use glucose more effectively instead of storing it as fat.

When I first wore a CGM early in my career as a precision nutritionist, it was a game-changer for how I understood my body's response to food. One of the most surprising lessons for me was how much more sensitive my body is to fructose compared to glucose. Being of Eastern European descent, my ancestors were never exposed to tropical fruits like mango, pineapple, and bananas, so I saw how these fruits would spike my blood sugar to as high as 180 mg/dL—much higher than what I'd see from eating a piece of sourdough bread.

This insight was shocking because we're so often told that fruit is a healthy snack. But for me, eating fruits alone—especially dried fruits—was not the best choice. The key lesson was to combine fruits with other foods to balance my blood sugar. Instead of snacking on watermelon by itself, I started pairing it with feta cheese in a Mediterranean cuisine salad. Mango became a topping for kale salads rather than a stand-alone treat, and I ate banana only in protein smoothies or with almond butter. These small adjustments helped me enjoy the foods I love without compromising my glucose levels, and they're lessons I now share with my clients.

Understanding how your body responds to specific foods isn't just enlightening—it's empowering. It's why I encourage everyone to try a CGM and discover their own unique glucose patterns. The insights can transform the way you approach food and help you make smarter, more balanced choices.

Here's why stabilizing blood sugar is essential:

- **Frequent glucose spikes** force your body to release large amounts of insulin, which over time can lead to insulin resistance—a precursor to type 2 diabetes, weight gain, and chronic inflammation.
- **High blood sugar levels** can damage blood vessels and nerves, increasing your risk of cardiovascular disease and other complications.
- **Balanced blood sugar** means more stable energy, reduced cravings, and better mood regulation, as glucose is the brain's primary fuel source.

Research shows that even small, consistent improvements in blood sugar control can significantly reduce the risk of metabolic disorders and improve overall health. For example, flattening glucose spikes not only protects against diabetes but also supports better digestion, immune function, and cognitive performance. The real-time feedback from a CGM is empowering. It takes the guesswork out of healthy eating and shows you how your unique body responds to your favorite foods. With this knowledge, you can make simple, impactful changes—like adjusting your meal composition, incorporating light movement after meals, or rethinking your snacking habits—to support stable energy levels, prevent metabolic issues, and live with vitality.

Pro Tip from a Dietitian

Start with a continuous glucose monitor (CGM) for fourteen to twenty-eight days. Traditionally, these devices required a prescription, as they were developed for people with diabetes and are typically only covered by insurance with a formal diagnosis. However, several companies—like Levels and Lingo—now make it easy to access a CGM without a doctor's prescription, offering programs designed for education, optimization, and prevention. Even without insurance, most pharmacies charge between seventy-five and ninety-nine dollars for a monitor, making it a relatively affordable tool for gaining insight into your metabolic health.

Treat it like an experiment: Test your favorite meals, snacks, and daily routines to see how your body responds. By the end of this trial, everything in this chapter will make so much more sense! Nothing beats the thirty-minute postmeal effect—when you see the numbers for yourself, it creates a whole new level of mind-body connection. You'll finally see what's happening beneath your skin and know exactly what steps to take. This deeper understanding of your body will empower you to keep your blood sugar stable, transforming your energy, focus, and overall health.

6. Testing for Food Sensitivities and Intolerances

Testing for food sensitivities and intolerances is a bit of a diagnostic gray area. While there is some disagreement among health professionals around the efficacy and use of food allergy and sensitivity testing, I am of the opinion that these tests can be very useful and even life-changing when interpreted properly.

It's an important way to understand if your diet is working for you, especially because food sensitivities (unlike allergies) have a delayed response. It can take hours or even days after eating an offending food for a reaction to occur. It is a cell-mediated response that occurs after food is eaten and then taken up by antigen-presenting cells, which are then exposed to immune cells and cause inflammation of pathways, and a wide range of symptoms that may affect various systems in the body, including the following:

- **Digestive symptoms**—diarrhea, constipation, abdominal bloating, gas, and nausea
- **Respiratory symptoms**—nasal congestion, chronic sinus infections, and postnasal drip
- **Musculoskeletal pain**—joint pain, muscle aches, and stiffness
- **Skin conditions**—eczema, acne, hives, rosacea, and other skin rashes
- **Neurological symptoms**—headaches, migraines, brain fog, and difficulty concentrating
- **Mood changes**—irritability, anxiety, and depression
- **Fatigue**—chronic tiredness and low energy levels
- **Immune system effects**—frequent colds, infections, or feeling run-down

The most common foods that cause problems are milk and wheat proteins, which is why so many people are embracing gluten- and dairy-free diets. Other big offenders include soy, corn, beans, eggs, nuts, shellfish, and the nightshade family (which includes tomatoes, peppers, potatoes, and eggplant).

Having lots of food sensitivities is a telltale sign of a leaky gut. Proteins are leaking into the bloodstream, causing an immune reaction and contributing to chronic inflammation. Fixing the gut fixes the sensitivities. I recommend bone broth, collagen, and glutamine supplements to my clients with many food sensitivities. This is why we take both a generalized and a personalized approach here, applying broader food and lifestyle principles for healing the gut while also eliminating the offending foods that are causing problems in the individual's system.

A food sensitivity panel completely changed the way I looked at food and started me on the road to finally healing my gut. Today, I recommend that my clients get a set of personalized data to find the root cause of their symptoms and create individualized nutrition recommendations.

Having lots of food sensitivities is a telltale sign of a leaky gut.

Food Allergies

IgE-Mediated Allergies

If you have a food allergy, you probably know about it! These are type 1 hypersensitivity reactions, commonly referred to as "true allergies." They involve an almost instant immune system response where immunoglobulin E (IgE) antibodies are produced in reaction to a specific food. This type of allergy can lead to immediate symptoms, such as hives, swelling, or even life-threatening anaphylaxis, occurring shortly after consuming the allergenic food.

Food Sensitivity and Intolerance

IgA/IgG (Gradual or Delayed) Type 2 Sensitivity

IgA and immunoglobulin G (IgG) are antibodies within the immune system, with IgG being the most prevalent antibody in the bloodstream. Unlike IgE-mediated allergies, IgA/IgG type 2 sensitivity reactions are delayed hypersensitivity responses. Symptoms may appear hours or even days after consuming an offending food, making it more challenging to pinpoint the cause.

These delayed reactions can result in various symptoms, often subtle or chronic, which might not be immediately associated with a specific food. Understanding these sensitivities is crucial for addressing underlying immune responses and improving overall well-being.

The most common foods I see causing problems are gluten and dairy. Others include eggs, corn, soy, grains, beans, and sometimes nightshades (tomatoes, peppers, potatoes, eggplant), nuts, and seeds.

Everyone has foods that cause symptoms for them. If you are experiencing recurring or chronic symptoms despite living a health-conscious lifestyle, you are very likely eating foods to which you are sensitive, intolerant, or even allergic.

Start with an Elimination Diet

My recommendation is to keep a food journal with your symptoms and start with an elimination diet. This simple, short-term diet is an effective way to learn how your body responds to things, and it saves a lot of money on more formal testing. If you're struggling with a persistent symptom and you don't know what might be causing or exacerbating it, this diet should be your first line of defense. Start here—it's going to give you a lot of insight and clarity.

Full disclosure: Elimination diets contain an element of restriction that some people might find difficult, boring, or distinctly unsexy. It may not appeal to your foodie sensibilities. As you know, I'm not about deprivation or focusing primarily on what you can't eat. The elimination diet is a temporary, short-term, and worthwhile exception to this approach, but it's really impactful. And it's worth dealing with the temporary annoyance of it because the return on investment is huge. Once you identify and avoid the foods that are causing you problems, you will free up so much energy and vitality to enjoy your life and appreciate the abundance of other foods that don't make you feel bad.

The elimination process is entirely driven by your symptoms. If you are having symptoms like bloating, eczema, allergies, fatigue, brain fog, or headaches, or if you've been diagnosed with an autoimmune condition, or even insomnia, anxiety, or depression, you may have hidden food sensitivities that are irritating your gut and contributing to chronic inflammation. These commonly include gluten, dairy, soy, beans, nightshades, eggs, sugar, shellfish, nuts, alcohol (especially wine and cocktails with added sugar), and caffeinated beverages. These are not problematic for everyone, but the key is to identify if they are a trigger for you.

The Elimination

Start by simply eliminating the three major trigger foods—gluten, dairy, and sugar—from your diet for twenty-one days. If you are aware of other foods that bother you, be sure to eliminate those also. During this time, refrain from eating processed foods and drinking alcohol and caffeinated beverages—this will support the process of clearing out your system. For twenty-one days, keep it simple and keep it clean. A good rule of thumb is to only eat something when you can tell what all the ingredients are (that means no mysterious sauces, frozen or prepared foods, or baked goods). This is the essence of the clean-eating approach, which means that what you see is what you get. For instance, you eat a piece of fish instead of a crab cake, which may contain wheat as a filler, or you have a steak instead of a burger. This will help retrain you to really understand what ingredients are in the foods you eat.

For the overachievers out there who are ready to go full-on in this process, you can also eliminate beans, nightshades, eggs, soy, corn, and nuts. However, I recommend just starting with the big three and going from there. This will be challenging enough already and will give you plenty of important data!

For these three weeks, plan ahead with your meals, minimize outings to restaurants and bars, and take the opportunity for a little extra rest and self-care.

Day 22: The reintroduction begins! Start by introducing one food at a time, taking two days for each food. You might start with gluten if you suspect that this is an issue for you. Gluten is a protein found in wheat, barley, and rye, commonly present in foods like bread, pasta, crackers, cereals, and baked goods. While you continue eating clean and following the diet, add a piece of bread or a bowl of pasta to one of your meals on day 22. Wait twenty-four hours and notice how you feel. If you're unsure, try it again the following day.

Day 23: Take note of any symptoms, both immediately after the meal and for the next forty-eight hours. (Often in the case of sensitivities, the reaction is delayed.) After two or three days, repeat the process with the next food, and the next, evaluating how you feel and logging any symptoms, until the process is complete.

My Elimination Diet Journey

The elimination diet is a lengthy process, but it is the gold standard for a personalized diet. When I first did my own elimination diet and food sensitivity panel with my dietitian, I ended up with what I call my "big no" list—no wheat, no dairy, no alcohol, no soy, no yeast, no nightshades . . . and on and on. After years of struggling with an imbalanced gut, my body was reacting to so many foods that it was depressing! I went cold turkey off all these foods. It wasn't easy, but after a week or so, I began to embrace it.

This was at the point in my journey where I'd already tried every diet and been to a multitude of GI doctors and dermatologists. I had gone to a dietitian on Madison Avenue in New York City who told me to measure my food and never to eat more than one tablespoon of almond butter. That was boring—I didn't like it. Finally I found the person who truly helped me. She worked with me to create a diet based on my body rather than philosophies. She said, "Here you go—this is what your body is telling you. Listen to it. Do something about it." She gave me the elimination diet to follow for three months, and I continued with a modified version of it for almost a year because it made me feel so much better.

During that time, I traveled all over—to St. Tropez, Las Vegas, London—and I was able to maintain the diet. Even though I had eliminated a number of foods, I discovered that there were still so many things I *could* eat, and that was where I focused my energy. I continued to have this personalized diet as a strong foundation to fall back on even as I went on with my life and enjoyed eating out and socializing over meals. I found that by eating this way 80 percent of the time and allowing myself to enjoy occasional indulgences the other 20 percent, I could still feel consistently energized, balanced, and in control of my health.

Don't forget: The end goal of this process is not only to discover the foods that your body loves but also to find a deeper and more sustainable pleasure from eating. As a bonus, eliminating certain foods in the long term can help to heal your gut so that you can actually enjoy a wider range of foods with minimal ill effects! If you discover you are sensitive to milk products, for instance, once you get your gut health back up to speed, you may find that you can mindfully enjoy dairy every now and again without feeling too terrible even if you no longer crave it daily .

If you end up heartbroken to find that something you love isn't working for you (au revoir, morning pain au chocolate!), please don't worry: There are always food solutions, which we explore in the next chapter. I make sure you're armed not only with healthier but still-delicious alternatives but also with rescue remedies to support your system if you decide to indulge in a trigger food. (This is okay every now and then as long as you're not truly allergic!) There's always something else that you can get excited about and focus on rather than on what you're giving up.

7. Hormonal Testing: Align Your Nutrition to Your Cycle

As women, our bodies are designed to shift throughout the month, and those changes affect everything—our energy, cravings, and even how we process food. Yet most nutrition advice ignores this reality, pushing one-size-fits-all plans that work better for men, who are hormonally consistent all month long. Learning to eat in sync with your cycle isn't just empowering; it's transformative.

Hormonal testing can reveal exactly how your levels of estrogen, progesterone, and other key hormones fluctuate, giving you the data to personalize your approach. Let's break it down into two key phases and how to make the most of them.

The Follicular Phase (Day 1 to Ovulation)

When your hormones are balanced at the start of your cycle, you naturally have more energy and mental clarity. This is the perfect time to experiment with your diet and incorporate practices like detoxing or fasting. During this phase,

- **Focus on detox-supporting foods** like broccoli and kale to help your liver process hormones.
- **Try a twelve- to fourteen-hour fasting window** to support cellular repair without stressing your body.
- **Explore lighter meals** with lean proteins, healthy fats, and vibrant vegetables.

A client of mine, Olivia, found that her energy and productivity soared when she swapped her usual carb-heavy breakfasts for nutrient-dense green smoothies and protein-rich salads during this phase.

The Luteal Phase (Postovulation to Menstruation)

After ovulation, progesterone rises, and your body begins preparing for a potential pregnancy. This hormonal shift can trigger increased hunger and cravings, especially for carbs and comfort foods. During this phase,

- Increase protein to stabilize blood sugar and support hormone production (think eggs, fish, or plant-based proteins).
- Add complex carbs like sweet potatoes or quinoa to fuel your body and ease cravings.
- Include magnesium-rich snacks like dark chocolate or pumpkin seeds to reduce bloating and irritability.

Samantha, another client, realized that she felt out of control during this phase, bingeing on sweets despite her usual healthy eating. By boosting her protein and magnesium intake during the luteal phase, she balanced her mood and reduced her cravings dramatically.

Why it matters: Trying to eat the same way all month long ignores your body's natural rhythm. Men can do it because their hormones are consistent, but as women, our needs change week to week. Embracing those changes isn't a weakness—it's a strategy for success.

- During the follicular phase, focus on detox and lighter meals.
- In the luteal phase, prioritize protein and complex carbs, and avoid restrictive diets.
- Use hormonal testing to understand your unique cycle and tailor your approach.

By aligning your nutrition with your cycle, you'll unlock more energy, balance cravings, and feel more in control. This isn't about restriction; it's about understanding your body and giving it what it needs when it needs it.

Learn from Your Bio-Individuality with the Right Tools

These seven tools—DNA methylation testing, comprehensive gut microbiome testing, advanced nutrient testing, fasting insulin testing, continuous glucose monitoring, observing food sensitivities and intolerances, and hormonal testing—offer a detailed understanding of your unique bio-individuality. With this data, you can create a highly personalized plan for your diet and nutrient intake, addressing your body's specific needs for optimal health and performance.

Understanding your biology isn't just about solving current health challenges—it's about building a foundation for long-term wellness and longevity. The you-tarian approach is all about customizing health and nutrition strategies that fit your individual body, and these tools are key to unlocking that path.

Most people won't need to test all seven areas at once. If you're navigating symptoms and looking for more clarity, start with the area that resonates most with your current experience. And remember: You don't have to do it alone. For those seeking more personalized support, I offer evaluation calls at gutbrainmethod.com, where we dive deeper into what your body truly needs to thrive.

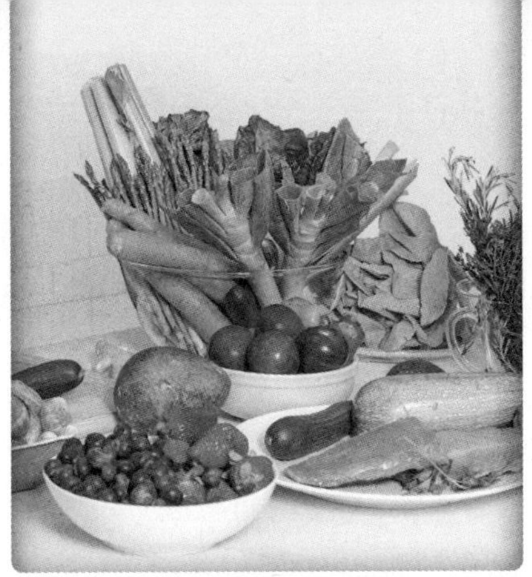

Chapter 4
Break Up with the Foods That Don't Love You: Reasons to Break Up

In the last chapter, you started to use observation and data gathering to figure out what foods your body does *not* love. Now we're going to look more closely at the foods that don't love you back. In addition to your personal trigger foods, a number of common inflammatory, gut-aggravating foods tend to create problems for most people, particularly when consumed in excess. These are the *foods that don't love you back*—and it's time for a conscious uncoupling.

I promise: This isn't going to be hard or depressing. I'm not about deprivation or hard nos. I'm a foodie but also a realist, so I want to be real about the fact that nobody is perfect all the time! And for many people, the pressure to restrict something from their diet 100 percent of the time is simply too difficult and quickly leads to feeling like a failure and giving up entirely. I advise my clients to follow the 80/20 rule: Eat clean, cook at home, and use nutrient-dense ingredients 80 percent of the time. The other 20 percent of the time, you can mindfully indulge without guilt in the foods that you love that are not quite so nutritious (even the things you know you can't tolerate, which are best avoided, but I help you manage the situation in case you end up overindulging). That's the equivalent of preparing a healthy, balanced meal at home on Monday, Tuesday, Wednesday, and Thursday, and then enjoying a meal out with friends on Friday night.

You might think you're just having a cookie, but at a cellular level you're triggering a cascade of effects that impact everything from your skin's collagen production to your brain's ability to focus. In my practice, I see the hidden damage of inflammatory foods show up in ways most people never connect to their diet: premature wrinkles, afternoon brain fog, unexplained fatigue, and that stubborn 3:00 PM energy crash.

Let's get specific about what's really happening inside your body when you consume inflammatory foods. That morning pastry isn't just empty calories—it's triggering advanced glycation end products (AGEs) that literally break down your skin's collagen, accelerating aging. That midafternoon soda or coffee isn't just a quick energy fix—it's damaging your mitochondria, the powerhouses of your cells, leading to fatigue that no amount of caffeine can fix.

The processed foods that dominate our modern diet do more than expand our waistlines—they're wreaking havoc at our most fundamental cellular level. Your mitochondria, those tiny energy factories in every cell, become less efficient with each assault of refined carbohydrates and trans fats. This doesn't just mean low energy; it means your brain can't fire properly (hello, brain fog), your skin can't repair itself effectively (welcome, premature aging), and your metabolism becomes increasingly compromised (hello, belly fat).

Foods That Don't Love You Back: Understanding Why Quality Matters

That warm, freshly baked croissant from your local bakery? Yes, it's still a treat worth enjoying occasionally. But the packaged croissant that's been sitting on a convenience store shelf for weeks? That's a different story entirely. Let me break down why quality matters and what's really happening in your body when you consume these foods.

Comfort Food Favorites

Your favorite drive-through burger combo isn't just a quick meal—it's a perfect storm of aging accelerators. The bun, made with refined flour and high-fructose corn syrup, triggers an immediate blood sugar spike that damages your mitochondria. The processed cheese, loaded with sodium caseinate and artificial preservatives, creates low-grade inflammation in your gut. The industrially produced beef, raised on antibiotics and inflammatory grain feed, lacks the beneficial omega-3s found in grass-fed meat. Each bite accelerates cellular aging through multiple pathways.

Here's my take as a foodie dietitian: If you're going to enjoy a burger, make it count. Choose a local restaurant using quality ingredients, or better yet, make it at home with grass-fed beef, a sourdough bun, and real aged cheese. This way, you'll satisfy your craving while minimizing cellular damage.

Caffeine

While one cup of coffee a day can be part of a healthy lifestyle, excessive caffeine intake from multiple sources can significantly impact your stress hormones and inflammation levels. Many people don't realize caffeine lurks in unexpected places beyond your morning coffee; it's found naturally in cocoa beans, guarana, and kola nuts. When my clients complain about anxiety or sleep issues, we often discover they're consuming caffeine throughout the day without realizing it—such as through coffee, energy drinks, pre-workout supplements, green tea, dark chocolate, or even certain medications and protein bars. My recommendation is to avoid drinking caffeinated beverages after 3:00 PM.

Energy Drinks and Popular Beverages: Beyond Empty Calories

That caramel Frappuccino you grab every morning? It's not just about the calories. The combination of industrial dairy, artificial caramel syrup, and refined sugar creates AGEs that break down your skin's collagen. Recent research shows these beverages can trigger intestinal permeability within just thirty minutes of consumption, leading to leaky gut.

Even more concerning are those zero-calorie energy drinks you might reach for during that afternoon slump. Don't be fooled by the sugar-free label. Artificial sweeteners like aspartame, sucralose, and acesulfame potassium have been shown to alter gut bacteria within hours of consumption, disrupting the delicate microbiome that governs everything from your mood to your metabolism. Studies reveal that these synthetic sweeteners can actually increase glucose intolerance, ironically making you more susceptible to diabetes and weight gain than regular sugar.

Those synthetic vitamins added to these drinks—such as folic acid instead of natural folate or synthetic B_{12}? Your body may process them differently. For example, some individuals with genetic variations might struggle to efficiently convert folic acid into its active form. Many of the amino acids in energy drinks, like taurine and carnitine, are lab creations. While these forms are generally bioavailable, their laboratory origin differs from the forms naturally found in whole foods. Excessive synthetic nutrients might interact with or mask deficiencies of their natural counterparts.

High caffeine content combined with artificial additives creates a double assault on your adrenal glands. That energy boost you feel? It's actually pushing your body into a stress response, flooding your system with cortisol and adrenaline. Over time, this can lead to adrenal fatigue, anxiety, and disrupted sleep patterns—creating a vicious cycle of needing more stimulants to get through the day.

Instead of saying never to your favorite drinks, become strategic. Choose high-quality coffee, such as single-origin, organic, or mold-free varieties like Purity Coffee, paired with organic milk—or learn to appreciate the complex flavors of plain espresso. If you need an energy boost, try mineral-rich coconut water or green tea, which contains L-theanine, which provides sustained energy without the crash. Save the sweeter drinks for true occasions rather than daily habits. When you do want something sweet, opt for naturally flavored sparkling water, brew your own herb-infused teas, or even make a quick fruit-infused water with slices of citrus or berries—simple, refreshing options that satisfy cravings without added sugar.

Snack Attack: The Cellular Impact

Those convenient bags of cheese puffs or pretzels in your pantry might seem harmless, but they're packed with acrylamides—compounds formed during high-temperature processing that directly damage your DNA and accelerate aging. The combination of refined carbs and industrial seed oils creates oxidative stress in your cells, essentially rusting them from the inside out.

My approach? Become a *qualitarian*—another term I developed to stress the importance of knowing the sources of your food. If you're craving something crunchy, opt for air-popped or stovetop popcorn made from whole kernels with real butter or olive oil—not the microwave bags loaded with additives—or grab a handful of raw or lightly roasted nuts. Save processed snacks for rare occasions, like a road trip, rather than making them a daily habit.

Restaurant Favorites: Making Smart Choices

That plate of fettuccine Alfredo from the Italian restaurant? The combination of industrial seed oils often used in sauces, along with refined pasta and conventional dairy products, can create a perfect storm of inflammation—especially in restaurants or packaged meals where high-quality ingredients are rarely guaranteed unless explicitly stated. Studies show that these combinations can impair your metabolic flexibility for up to seventy-two hours after eating.

But this doesn't mean never enjoying pasta again. Choose restaurants that make sauces from scratch using real, whole ingredients—and don't hesitate to call ahead and ask. At home, learn to make your own sauces using extra virgin, cold-pressed olive oil, fresh organic cream, and authentic Parmigiano-Reggiano for rich flavor and nutrient density. The difference isn't just in the taste—it's in how your body processes these real ingredients.

Remember: The goal isn't perfection but becoming a qualitarian. Choose high-quality, minimally processed foods 80 percent of the time. For the other 20 percent, when you do indulge in foods that don't love you back, make sure they're worth it. Choose quality versions of your favorites rather than processed alternatives.

Here's what to avoid and limit on a daily basis to create a healthier body and prevent issues with digestion, metabolism, and blood sugar. What do these foods have in common? They all spike your blood sugar levels and cause inflammation—the number-one cause of most diseases. To unlock healthy metabolism and overall health, we want to keep our insulin levels low and reduce inflammation.

Foods That Cause Inflammation

Try to avoid or minimize these foods as much as possible:

- **Refined carbohydrates,** such as white bread, pastries, and most packaged baked goods
- **Sugar-sweetened snacks,** including candy, cookies, and sweetened granola bars
- **Fried foods,** especially those from fast-food restaurants or prepackaged frozen meals
- **Sugary beverages,** like soda, energy drinks, and sweetened teas
- **Processed meats**, such as hot dogs, sausage, deli meats, and cold cuts—particularly those with added preservatives, nitrates, or excess sodium
- **Margarine, shortening, and products containing trans fats,** which can promote inflammation and increase cardiovascular risk

If you want to support your metabolism, skin, and hormone balance, you'll want to steer clear of certain foods and drinks.

Sugar

When reducing or eliminating sugar-containing foods, remember that sugar is both physiologically and psychologically addictive, and it takes time (approximately three to four weeks) to build a new level of tolerance. Most of my clients notice how their "taste buds change" as they consume less sugar, and after a while, most of the sugary treats taste far too sweet. I encourage you to give a sugar detox a try at least once to learn about how cravings work and the flexibility of your taste buds.

How Sugar Disrupts Your Body: Six Key Influencers

1. **Metabolism.** Constant blood sugar spikes lead to insulin resistance, which slows down your metabolism and makes weight management more difficult over time.
2. **Skin.** Sugar triggers glycation, a chemical process that damages collagen and elastin, the proteins responsible for skin's firmness and elasticity. The result? Premature aging, dullness, and fine lines.
3. **Hormones.** Excess sugar disrupts insulin regulation, which can throw off other hormones like cortisol, estrogen, and progesterone, leading to mood swings, fatigue, and cycle irregularities.
4. **Gut health.** Sugar and artificial sweeteners like Splenda, sorbitol, and xylitol can wreak havoc on your gut microbiome. These compounds may increase fecal pH, reduce beneficial bacteria, and trigger digestive symptoms such as gas, cramps,

and diarrhea. Choose natural, whole-food sweeteners like raw honey or blackstrap molasses when needed.

5. **Sugar consumption habits.** To reduce inflammation and support gut and metabolic health, eliminate added sugars and minimize even natural sugars like those found in melons and mangoes. Sugar fuels bacterial overgrowth and is a major contributor to bloating and GI distress. Focus on a plant-forward, whole-food diet with limited processed snacks, desserts, and sugar-laden beverages.
6. **Alcohol.** Alcohol, especially beer and sweet cocktails—acts like liquid sugar in the body. It can increase inflammation, spike blood sugar, and negatively impact your gut microbiome, worsening symptoms like bloating, fatigue, and skin flare-ups.

The Truth About Alcohol: A Dietitian's Guide

Let me be real about alcohol—as someone who appreciates a good glass of wine but also knows exactly what it does to our bodies. Those fancy cocktails at your favorite bar? They're often sugar bombs in disguise. A typical mojito contains two to three pumps of simple syrup plus sugary lime cordial, while a margarita mix can pack more sugar than a candy bar. Even those "healthy" skinny cocktails often contain artificial sweeteners that can disrupt your gut microbiome.

Here's what really happens in your body when you drink:

Metabolism mayhem. Alcohol hits your liver like a metabolic pause button. While your liver is busy processing ethanol (it prioritizes this over everything else), all fat burning comes to a screeching halt. That late-night pizza after drinking? It's going straight to storage because your liver is too busy dealing with the alcohol to properly metabolize anything else.

Accelerated skin aging. Within hours of drinking, alcohol pulls water from your skin cells, leading to that puffy, dehydrated look the next morning. Ever notice those tiny red blood vessels becoming more visible? That's because alcohol dilates your blood vessels, potentially triggering or worsening rosacea. For my clients focused on antiaging, I explain how regular drinking can accelerate collagen breakdown, leading to premature wrinkles.

Hormone havoc. Here's what most people don't realize: Alcohol throws your entire hormonal system into chaos. Your liver—which should be breaking down excess estrogen—becomes too preoccupied with alcohol to do its job properly. This can lead to estrogen dominance, especially in women, causing everything from mood swings to stubborn belly fat.

Pro Tip from a Dietitian

When at social events, I order sparkling water with lime in a wine glass or create my own "cocktail" with kombucha and fresh citrus. Nobody needs to know you're not drinking, and you'll feel amazing the next day!

Mindful Drinking Strategies

Here's my biggest lesson from years of working with clients (and my own experience): If you're going to drink alcohol, *how* you drink matters as much as *what* you drink.

Start with sixteen ounces of water before your first drink. When alcohol hits an empty stomach, ethanol is absorbed rapidly into your bloodstream and crosses the blood-brain barrier like a bullet train—that's why you can feel tipsy so quickly when drinking before dinner.

The science is clear: Consuming alcohol with food, especially a combination of fiber, protein, and healthy fats, can slow ethanol absorption by up to 50 percent.

Follow each alcoholic beverage with eight to twelve ounces of water, and add electrolytes to your water if you have more than two drinks.

My Protocol for Smarter Drinking

If you're going to drink, here's how to do it with minimal damage:

- Never drink on an empty stomach: Always eat a meal containing fiber, protein, and healthy fats first (like salmon with quinoa and avocado).
- Take B-complex vitamins before drinking (alcohol depletes B vitamins).
- Choose your drinks wisely: Go for clear spirits (vodka, tequila) with sparkling water and fresh citrus over sugary cocktails, sweet wines, and beer (liquid bread).
- Consider a moderate choice: Try dry red wine, which contains resveratrol, an antioxidant.
- Hydrate aggressively: Alternate each alcoholic drink with eight to twelve ounces of water.
- Support your liver: Include cruciferous vegetables in your pre-drinking meal (broccoli, cauliflower, Brussels sprouts) to boost detoxification pathways.
- Stop drinking three to four hours before bedtime for better sleep quality.

The science behind hangover prevention is fascinating: Alcohol is a diuretic that depletes essential minerals and B vitamins. By staying hydrated and eating nutrient-dense foods before drinking, you're giving your body the resources it needs to process alcohol more efficiently.

Remember: This isn't about encouraging drinking. It's about being realistic and strategic by using tools for harm reduction when you do choose to indulge. Your body will thank you the next morning.

To support your body, choose quality over quantity, and always have a plan to support your body's detox pathways. Some additional tips:

- Support your liver's detoxification pathways with strategic supplementation. Milk thistle *(Silybum marianum)* contains silymarin, a powerful flavonoid complex that's been shown in clinical studies to protect liver cells from alcohol-induced oxidative stress and enhance glutathione production—your body's master antioxidant. This is especially important because alcohol depletes glutathione stores, leaving the liver more vulnerable to damage. For general liver support, most studies use 200 to 400 mg of silymarin per day, but always consult a healthcare provider for personalized guidance.
- Activated charcoal works through a process called adsorption (not absorption), binding to toxins and preventing their absorption in your gut. It's commonly available in capsule or tablet form, and a typical dose ranges from 250 to 500 mg; taking it thirty minutes before drinking can help bind to congeners—the toxic byproducts in alcohol that contribute to hangovers. However, timing is crucial: Take it too close to drinking, and it might bind to nutrients from your protective pre-drinking meal. I recommend taking it at the end of your night or the next morning to help clear remaining toxins but never with other medications or supplements as it can bind to those also.

Caffeine

- **Metabolism.** While caffeine can temporarily boost metabolism, excessive intake can lead to adrenal fatigue, making your metabolism sluggish over time.
- **Skin.** Too much caffeine can dehydrate the skin and exacerbate conditions like acne and inflammation.
- **Hormones.** Caffeine can increase cortisol levels, leading to stress-related hormonal imbalances and disruptions in sleep, which is crucial for hormone regulation.

Processed and Packaged Foods

- **Metabolism.** These foods are often high in unhealthy fats, sugars, and additives that disrupt your metabolism and promote fat storage.
- **Skin.** Processed foods can cause inflammation, leading to breakouts, redness, and uneven skin tone.
- **Hormones.** Artificial ingredients and preservatives can interfere with your endocrine system, affecting hormone production and balance.

Fried Food

- **Metabolism.** Fried food is high in trans fats, which are known to slow down metabolism and increase the risk of obesity.
- **Skin.** These fats promote inflammation and oxidative stress, leading to breakouts and premature aging.
- **Hormones.** Fried foods can disrupt hormonal balance by affecting insulin sensitivity and increasing levels of unhealthy fats in the body.

Gluten and Dairy

I'm focusing on gluten and dairy too but for reasons that have nothing to do with the fact that going gluten-free and drinking oat milk are currently trendy (and I actually don't recommend oat milk, but we get into that later). More and more people are going gluten- and dairy-free for good reason. If you struggle with any degree of gut imbalance (which most people do!), these foods will create a negative reaction. Here's the short version of the story: An abundance of research shows that gluten, dairy, and sugar disrupt the composition of gut microbiota and lead to increased intestinal permeability (aka the dreaded leaky gut). Wheat and milk proteins leak out of the intestines and into the bloodstream, where they create an inflammatory reaction. Gluten may be the biggest offender when it comes to leaky gut. Research has shown that gluten is one of the main drivers of zonulin, which regulates intestinal permeability. Zonulin signals the lining of the gut to open up and make those gaps so that food particles are able to cross over into the bloodstream. Gluten expert Dr. Alessio Fasano at Harvard has found that gluten triggers an increase in zonulin not only in people who are gluten-intolerant or with celiac disease but in *everyone.*

Conventional Dairy

- **Metabolism.** Can lead to inflammation and digestive issues, slowing down your metabolic rate.
- **Skin.** Dairy is a common trigger for acne and other skin conditions due to hormones and inflammatory proteins.
- **Hormones.** Conventional dairy often contains added hormones, which can disrupt your own hormone balance, leading to issues like estrogen dominance.

Genetically Modified (GMO) Gluten

- **Metabolism.** GMO gluten can cause digestive distress and inflammation, which can hinder metabolic function.
- **Skin.** For those sensitive to gluten, it can trigger skin conditions like eczema and psoriasis.
- **Hormones.** Gluten sensitivity can lead to systemic inflammation, affecting thyroid function and overall hormone balance.

GMO Soy

- **Metabolism.** GMO soy can interfere with thyroid function, which directly impacts metabolic rate.
- **Skin.** Soy can mimic estrogen in the body, potentially leading to skin issues like acne and hyperpigmentation.
- **Hormones.** The phytoestrogens in soy can disrupt hormonal balance, especially for those prone to estrogen-related conditions.

Meat Alternatives ("Fake Anything" Food)

- **Metabolism.** Highly processed meat alternatives often contain additives, fillers, and unhealthy fats that can slow down your metabolism.
- **Skin.** These products can cause inflammation and irritation, negatively impacting skin health.
- **Hormones.** The additives and synthetic ingredients can interfere with natural hormone production and balance, leading to issues like increased cortisol or disrupted estrogen levels.

By avoiding these foods and focusing on a diet rich in whole, natural ingredients, you'll be supporting your metabolism, improving your skin, and keeping your hormones balanced.

When You Eat Matters as Much as What You Eat

You just finished a long day at work, had a light dinner at 6:00 PM, and now it's 9:30 PM. You're curled up on the couch, bingeing your favorite Netflix series, and those late-night munchies start creeping in. I see this pattern constantly with my high-performing, busy clients—that evening snacky feeling that has nothing to do with actual hunger and everything to do with habit.

Let me share a story about my client Maria. She came to me frustrated about her stubborn belly fat despite eating clean and exercising regularly. Her issue wasn't what she was eating—it was when. Like many busy professionals, she'd eat a small breakfast, rush through lunch, and then backload her calories into the evening, often snacking right up until bedtime. Her body never had a chance to tap into fat burning during sleep because it was too busy digesting that 10:00 PM bowl of "healthy" cereal.

Here's what I taught Maria, and what I'm teaching you now: *Frontloading your calories earlier in the day and avoiding food three to four hours before sleep is one of the most powerful tools in the Foodie Diet protocol.* I've seen firsthand how this approach—when done properly—can be life-changing for weight loss, better energy in the morning, and sleep quality.

Within weeks of implementing this change, Maria woke up actually feeling hungry for breakfast (a sign of a healthy metabolism), her sleep quality improved dramatically, and yes, her waistline began to slim down. Best of all, her energy levels soared because she was finally giving her body the nighttime break it needed for cellular repair.

Simplicity in Practice: Start with Intermittent Fasting

You don't have to jump into extreme fasting to see the benefits. A simple way to start is with *intermittent fasting*—fasting for twelve to sixteen hours overnight and eating during an eight- to twelve-hour window during the day. This schedule gives your body the rest it needs to activate autophagy (a process where your body removes damaged cells and regenerates healthier ones) and promote gut healing without feeling deprived.

Pro Tip from a Dietitian

Start with a twelve-hour fasting window. For example, if you finish dinner at 6:00 PM, don't eat again until 6:00 the next day. During your fasting window, stay hydrated with water, electrolyte-balanced fluids, herbal teas, or green tea, which also provides antioxidants to support overall health.

Once you feel comfortable, you can gradually extend your fasting period to fourteen to sixteen hours, five to six days a week. That said, what may be even more important than the fasting window itself is not eating for at least three to four hours before bedtime. Research on circadian rhythms and metabolism shows that late-night eating can disrupt sleep, impair digestion, and spike overnight blood sugar, even if your overall fasting period is technically long enough.

So, if you typically finish dinner around 7:30 PM and go to bed at 11:00 to 11:30 PM, you're on the right track. The goal isn't perfection but rhythm and consistency. When late-night cravings hit, sip on herbal tea or sparkling water instead. Your morning self will thank you with a flatter belly, clearer mind, and more vibrant energy.

My personal mindset trick? Don't focus on restriction. Instead, think of it as eating with elegance and mindfulness, especially when breaking the fast. When your brain is seeking a reward, avoid reaching for sugary or heavy meals. Your gut and hormones will thank you.

Fasting is a great way to hit the reset button and renegotiate your relationship with food.

Benefits of Fasting

The science behind fasting is fascinating. When you avoid late-night eating and create a proper fasting window, you trigger autophagy—a cellular cleanup process where your body removes damaged cells and regenerates healthier ones. Think of it as your body's nightly maintenance crew that only shows up when the kitchen is closed.

Autophagy: Fasting's Cellular Housekeeping

One of the most exciting benefits of fasting is its ability to trigger autophagy, when your body gets rid of old, dysfunctional cells to make room for new, vibrant ones. This process is crucial for reducing oxidative stress, lowering inflammation, and supporting overall cellular health.

Autophagy helps prevent cellular senescence (the state where cells stop dividing and start accumulating), which is one of the key drivers of aging. By promoting cellular repair, fasting may help slow the aging process and support long-term health.

Gut Health Reset

Fasting allows your digestive system to take a much-needed break. In a world where we often eat late into the night, our gut rarely gets the rest it needs to heal and repair. Fasting helps reduce inflammation and gives your gut time to restore intestinal permeability—that is, to heal your leaky gut.

When you fast, you also help balance your gut microbiota. This community of bacteria, fungi, and other microorganisms plays a vital role in digestion, immune function, and even mental health. Fasting can lead to an increase in beneficial bacteria, supporting a healthier microbiome, better digestion, and more efficient nutrient absorption.

Blood Sugar and Metabolic Health: Stabilizing the Foundation

Fasting has profound effects on insulin sensitivity and blood sugar regulation. Insulin resistance is one of the major culprits behind metabolic disorders like diabetes, weight gain, and even heart disease. By fasting, you give your body a chance to stabilize insulin levels, which helps regulate blood sugar and improve metabolic function.

Fasting also encourages your body to switch from burning glucose (sugar) to burning fat for energy—a process known as lipid metabolism. This shift not only helps with weight management but also promotes fat-burning and energy balance, which is key for long-term health and longevity.

Fasting for Longevity and Gut Health: Is It for Everyone?

While fasting has many benefits, it's not a one-size-fits-all solution. For some people, particularly those with certain medical conditions or who are pregnant, fasting may not be appropriate. If you're considering fasting, it's important to consult with a healthcare provider or dietitian to make sure it's safe for you and to create a fasting plan that fits your individual needs.

Post-Fasting: Prioritize Gut-Friendly Foods

How you break your fast is just as important as the fast itself. After fasting, it's essential to nourish your body with foods that support gut health and reduce inflammation. Focus on prebiotic-rich and anti-inflammatory foods that promote microbial diversity and healing.

Here are some great options to break your fast:

- **Nonstarchy vegetables:** spinach, kale, zucchini, cucumber, arugula, bell peppers
- **Healthy fats:** avocado, olive oil, ghee, tahini, chia seeds, flaxseeds
- **Lean proteins:** salmon, chicken, eggs, or plant-based options like tofu, tempeh, or lentils
- **Fermented foods:** kimchi, sauerkraut, unsweetened yogurt, kefir, or miso

These foods help replenish your gut microbiome, support nutrient absorption, and give your body the nutrients it needs after a period of fasting.

Less Is More: Fasting for a Healthier, Longer Life

Fasting can be a powerful tool for both longevity and gut health. It activates your body's natural repair systems through autophagy, helps your gut reset and heal, and supports metabolic health by improving insulin sensitivity and encouraging fat burning. By starting with intermittent fasting and focusing on gut-friendly foods post-fast, you can harness the power of fasting to boost your overall health and vitality.

Now that we've cleared the pathway by identifying the foods that don't serve your health and understanding the power of when you eat, it's time to get excited. This is where the real magic of the Foodie Diet begins: meeting the MVPs, our most valuable players in the nutrition game.

In the next chapter, we explore the foods that will love you back, supporting your vitality, longevity, and—yes—your joy in eating. Because remember: Being a qualitarian and a you-tarian isn't about restriction; it's about choosing foods that serve both your health and your happiness.

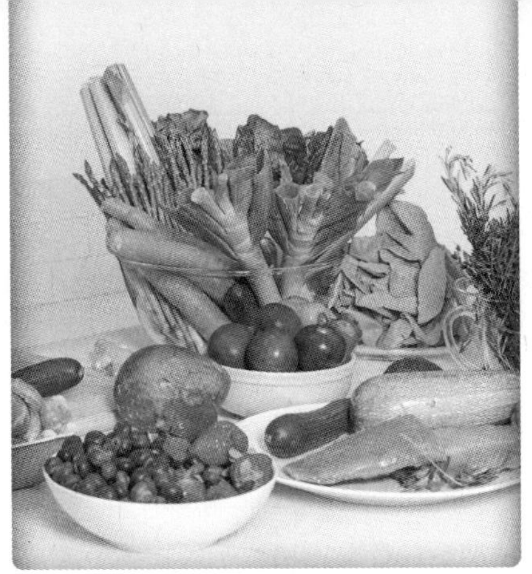

Chapter 5

Love the Foods That Love You Back: Food Groups, Superfoods, and Antioxidants

As a dietitian who loves food and believes in the power of eating well, I'm here to show you that a healthy diet doesn't mean giving up on flavor, joy, or indulgence. It's about balance, variety, and knowing what works best for your body. In this chapter, we'll explore the essential building blocks of a gut-friendly, longevity-focused diet, from proteins, fats, and carbohydrates to advanced compounds like shilajit, spirulina, and elderberry. You'll also discover how to enjoy foods like steak, bread, and butter without guilt, making them part of a sustainable lifestyle.

Let's cut through the noise about what you should and shouldn't eat. After years of working with clients and experiencing my own journey with food, I've learned that nutrition isn't about restriction—it's about understanding how different foods serve your body and choosing the ones that make you thrive.

Before we dive into the exciting world of antioxidants and superfoods, let's get crystal clear about the three fundamental building blocks of nutrition: proteins, fats, and carbohydrates. I find that once my clients truly understand these basics, everything else falls into place naturally.

The Three Major Food Groups: Proteins, Fats, and Carbohydrates

Think of these three macronutrients as your body's primary language. Just like you need different words to express yourself clearly, your body needs various forms of each macronutrient to function optimally. The quality of these words matters—there's a world of difference between the protein in a grass-fed steak and a processed protein bar, between the fats in an avocado and those in a bag of chips, between the carbohydrates in a sweet potato and a sugary cereal.

In my practice, I've seen how understanding these fundamentals transforms people's relationship with food. Suddenly, that piece of sourdough bread isn't bad—it's a source of complex carbohydrates that can feed your gut bacteria. That grass-fed steak isn't a guilty pleasure—it's a concentrated source of nutrients your body recognizes and knows how to use.

Let's explore how each of these food groups can work for you, not against you, as we build a foundation for understanding the more advanced nutrients that will help you optimize your health and longevity.

When you approach food with mindfulness and understanding, it becomes your most powerful ally for gut health, energy, and long-term vitality. Let's dive into the abundance of options you should know about and enjoy.

Everyone Loves Protein

Proteins are the foundation of a healthy diet and are essential for building and repairing tissues, supporting immune function, and maintaining muscle mass as we age.

As a functional medicine dietitian, I've seen firsthand how optimizing protein intake can transform health, particularly as we age. The old RDA (recommended dietary allowance) of 0.8 g of protein per kilogram of body weight is just the minimum to prevent deficiency—not what we need for optimal health and longevity.

Leading longevity experts, including Dr. Rhonda Patrick and Dr. Gabrielle Lyon, are redefining what a healthy portion of protein is while emphasizing the importance of optimal protein intake—not just for fitness and strength but as a cornerstone of overall health and longevity to increase muscle strength and reduce frailty.

In my practice, I recommend different protein targets based on life stage and goals. For my clients over age forty, I often suggest 1.2 to 1.6 g of protein per kilogram of body weight to combat the natural loss of muscle mass that occurs with aging. For my athletic clients or those in recovery **after an intense athletic event,** we might go up to 2 g per kilogram to support tissue repair and maintain lean muscle mass.

As we age, the body naturally loses muscle mass, a process known as *sarcopenia*, which can lead to reduced strength, mobility, and metabolic health. In her book *Forever Strong*, Dr. Gabrielle Lyon calls muscle the "organ of longevity," highlighting how maintaining and building lean muscle mass is key to reducing inflammation, supporting metabolism, and enhancing overall quality of life. To prevent muscle loss and optimize health, adequate protein intake is nonnegotiable.

Science backs this up. Recent research from leading longevity experts confirms what I've observed clinically: Higher protein intake, particularly from high-quality sources, is crucial not just for muscle maintenance but for immune function, cognitive health, and metabolic efficiency. This isn't just about building muscle—it's about maintaining the structural integrity of every cell in your body.

Research suggests that optimal protein intake is higher than the standard dietary recommendations for many people, especially for active adults over forty who exercise regularly. Dr. Lyon advocates for a minimum of 1.6 to 2.2 g of protein per kilogram of body weight daily, with a focus on quality protein sources. This translates to about 100 to 150 g of protein daily for an individual weighing 150 pounds (68 kg). My recommendation is to *distribute protein intake evenly across meals to maximize muscle protein synthesis, particularly in older adults.*

High-quality protein sources include grass-fed beef and pasture-raised poultry, which provide complete proteins rich in all nine essential amino acids necessary for muscle repair and immune support. They're also a good source of iron and zinc. Wild-caught fish, such as salmon, mackerel, and sardines, offer not only high-quality protein but also omega-3 fatty acids, which reduce inflammation and support brain and heart health. Eggs are another excellent, cost-effective source of high-quality protein and choline, which supports brain health and liver function. For vegetarians and vegans, complete protein can be found in tofu, tempeh, edamame, quinoa, buckwheat, and hemp seeds. While many plant proteins are incomplete on their own, combining foods like legumes and whole grains (e.g., rice and beans) can provide a full amino acid profile. Spirulina, nutritional yeast, and protein powders made from peas, brown rice, or hemp can also help meet daily protein needs—especially when paired strategically throughout the day.

Pro Tip from a Dietitian

Timing matters as much as quantity. I guide my clients to spread their protein intake throughout the day rather than loading up at dinner, which is what most Americans do. Your body can optimally utilize about 20 to 40 g of protein per meal for muscle protein synthesis. Think of it as opening a savings account for your muscles—regular deposits throughout the day add up and are more effective than one large dump done sporadically.

Remember, protein needs are highly individual and depend on your size, activity level, age, and current weight. While a sedentary office worker might need just 1 g per kilogram of body weight, an active fifty-year-old woman trying to maintain muscle mass might need 1.6 g per kilogram. And here's something many people don't realize: Protein isn't a "free" food. At 4 calories per gram, excessive protein intake can contribute to weight gain just like any other macronutrient. I've seen clients overdo protein, thinking it can't impact their weight, only to find their progress stalling because of the extra calories.

Understanding Protein Bioavailability: Animal Versus Plant Sources

Before we dive into specific plant proteins, let's address a crucial distinction in protein quality that I discuss with all my clients. Animal proteins are considered "complete" proteins because they contain all nine essential amino acids in optimal ratios that your body can readily use. Their bioavailability—meaning how efficiently your body can absorb and utilize them—typically ranges from 90 to 100 percent.

Plant proteins, while valuable, often have lower bioavailability (ranging from 60 to 80 percent) and may be missing or low in certain essential amino acids. This doesn't mean they're inferior—it just means we need to be strategic about combining them. Ancient grains like quinoa and buckwheat are unique in the plant world because they contain all essential amino acids, though in different ratios than animal proteins.

This is why I often discuss amino acid complementarity with my plant-based clients. For example, when you combine rice with legumes, you're creating a complete protein profile because each compensates for what the other lacks. Understanding this helps explain why traditional food cultures often intuitively paired these foods together.

The Essential Nine: Amino Acid Building Blocks

Your body requires nine essential amino acids that it cannot produce on its own, and understanding each one's role can revolutionize how you approach protein recommendation. Let me break down these critical building blocks and their impact on your health:

Leucine, isoleucine, and valine—known as branched-chain amino acids (BCAAs)—are crucial for muscle protein synthesis and energy production. Leucine, in particular, acts as a metabolic trigger for muscle growth and repair. I've seen clients struggling with postexercise recovery and muscle maintenance simply because they weren't getting enough leucine in their diet. While BCAA supplements are popular in fitness circles, you can obtain optimal amounts from whole food sources like grass-fed meat, wild-caught fish, and eggs if consumed daily.

Lysine, often deficient in plant-based diets, is essential for collagen formation, immune function, and calcium absorption. A lysine deficiency can manifest as fatigue, slow wound healing, and even recurring cold sores. This is why I pay special attention to lysine intake with my vegan clients and recommend extra supplementation during physical and emotional stress, as well as during traveling, to support the immune system.

Methionine and threonine support liver detoxification pathways. Methionine is particularly interesting because it's crucial for the production of glutathione, your body's master antioxidant. When clients show signs of poor detoxification, I recommend not only an extra load of green vegetables but often trace it back to insufficient methionine intake from plant and animal protein sources.

Phenylalanine and tryptophan are precursors to neurotransmitters that regulate mood, sleep, and appetite. Tryptophan converts to serotonin, while phenylalanine becomes tyrosine, then dopamine. Serotonin is the neurotransmitter responsible for good mood originating in the gut, which explains why protein deficiency can impact mental health and sleep quality significantly.

While sometimes overlooked, histidine is crucial for hemoglobin synthesis, healthy insulin, and tissue repair. Recent research shows histidine's role in protecting against oxidative stress and supporting cognitive function. I've noticed that athletes and highly active individuals often need more histidine than sedentary people due to higher muscle mass.

Pro Tip from a Dietitian

While supplementation might be necessary in specific cases, I always recommend getting these amino acids from whole food sources first. The synergistic effects of consuming complete protein sources with fiber and healthy fats cannot be replicated by individual amino acid supplements.

The Power of Plant Proteins

Plant proteins do double duty in your body. Take lentils and beans, for example. Recent studies from the American Gut Project at the University of California, San Diego, show that just one serving provides not only protein but also resistant starch and fiber that specifically feed *Bifidobacterium* and *Lactobacillus*—key bacterial species for gut health. In my practice, I've seen dramatic improvements in digestive health when clients incorporate these foods regularly.

Quinoa stands out as particularly interesting. While most plant proteins are incomplete, quinoa provides all nine essential amino acids in ratios similar to animal protein. Research published in the journal *Nutrients* shows that quinoa's unique amino acid profile, combined with its prebiotic compounds, supports both protein synthesis and gut barrier function. Like quinoa, buckwheat is another ancient grain that deserves special attention. Despite its name, buckwheat isn't related to wheat at all—it's actually a seed from the rhubarb family. What makes buckwheat particularly fascinating is its own unique amino acid profile, especially high in lysine and arginine, amino acids often lacking in other plant-based foods. Recent research shows that buckwheat's content of rutin—a powerful flavonoid—supports cardiovascular health by improving blood vessel flexibility and reducing inflammation.

In my practice, I often recommend buckwheat to clients looking for gluten-free alternatives that pack a real nutritional punch. Its resistant starch content feeds beneficial gut bacteria while its high magnesium levels support muscle recovery and sleep quality. As a bonus, buckwheat's prebiotic fibers help establish a diverse microbiome, which we now know is crucial for everything from immune function to mental health.

A Foodie Guide to Beans

I love recommending beans and legumes to my clients because only 5 percent of Americans are getting enough fiber in their diet and beans are nutrient-dense foods that are delicious, high in plant-based proteins, and also high in gut-microbiome-supporting fiber. Research from the Harvard School of Public Health demonstrates that legume consumption significantly reduces cardiovascular disease risk and improves metabolic health. The specific amino acid profiles and fiber content of different beans offer unique benefits worthy of understanding. Of course, ideally, I recommend buying them from small farms like Rancho Gordo in California, where they truly care about how they treat their products and the soil, which enhances the nutrient density of the produce.

Let me break down the science behind each variety of beans:

- **Adzuki beans** hold a special place in my functional medicine practice for their exceptional therapeutic properties. These small red beans, revered in Japanese medicine, pack the highest antioxidant punch among legumes, as well as fiber for gut health. For optimal benefits, I recommend cooking them with kombu seaweed and combining with black sesame seeds—a preparation method that maximizes nutrient absorption and digestibility. Start with a ¼-cup serving twice weekly, especially during detoxification protocols, and notice how your body responds to this ancient healing food. An adzuki bean salad recipe appears in Chapter 9.

- **Chickpeas** (garbanzo beans) contain a unique fiber profile that specifically feeds *Akkermansia muciniphila*, a beneficial gut bacteria associated with improved metabolic health. Clinical studies show that their unique carbohydrate structure helps stabilize blood sugar more effectively than other legumes.
- **Black beans** provide specific anthocyanins that cross the blood-brain barrier, with research showing potential neuroprotective benefits. Their resistant starch content promotes butyrate production, supporting gut barrier function.
- **White beans** (cannellini and great northern) contain the highest levels of alpha-amylase inhibitors among legumes, helping regulate postmeal blood sugar spikes. In my practice, I often recommend these varieties to clients monitoring their glucose levels.

Pro Tip from a Dietitian

For optimal nutrient absorption and reduced digestive discomfort, I recommend soaking all dried beans for twenty-four hours with a strip of kombu seaweed. This traditional practice is supported by research showing up to 60 percent reduction in oligosaccharides that can cause bloating. Also, don't miss the viral Dense Bean Salad recipe in Chapter 9, a delicious and nourishing way to enjoy gut-friendly beans!

Fiber-Rich Plant Protein Powerhouses

As a dietitian who focuses on both nutrient density and gut health, I recommend the most beneficial plant-based protein sources that deliver a *dual benefit of protein and fiber*—something you won't find in animal proteins. Here's what I recommend to my clients who want to optimize both their protein intake and gut health.

Legumes lead the pack. A cup of lentils provides 18 g of protein and 15 g of fiber, making them one of nature's most perfect foods for gut health and sustained energy. Black beans come in strong with 15 g of protein and 15 g of fiber per cup, while chickpeas offer 14 g of protein and 12 g of fiber, along with resistant starch that feeds beneficial gut bacteria.

Ancient grains deserve special attention. Quinoa packs 8 g of complete protein and 5 g of fiber per cup, while buckwheat offers 6 g of protein and 4.5 g of fiber. Both contain prebiotic fibers that support microbiome diversity. Tempeh and edamame, both whole soy foods, provide, respectively, 31 g and 17 g of protein per cup, along with 10 g and 8 g of fiber. Unlike processed soy products, these traditional forms offer intact fiber matrices that support gut health. Tofu, while still a good plant-based protein source (around 20 g per cup), is lower in fiber due to its processing. It's still a valuable option in a gut-healthy diet, especially when paired with fiber-rich vegetables and fermented foods.

Pro Tip from a Dietitian

Aim for adding plant-based proteins to your diet at least two to three times a week or having a vegetarian detox day once a week. Combine these foods for maximum benefit. For example, I recommend a bowl of quinoa with lentils and edamame for a complete protein profile plus diverse fiber sources that support different beneficial gut bacteria strains.

Collagen, the Most Abundant Protein in the Human Body

Now let's talk about collagen—a protein that's become a buzzword but is often misunderstood. Clinical studies show that collagen isn't just about skin beauty; it provides specific amino acids (glycine, proline, and hydroxyproline) that act as building blocks for your intestinal lining. This is why I often recommend bone broth to my clients with gut permeability issues.

Here's what the research reveals about collagen's benefits:

- Supports gut barrier integrity through specific peptides that help rebuild the intestinal lining.
- Provides glycine, which reduces inflammation and supports detoxification.
- Contains proline, essential for wound healing and tissue repair.

Pro Tip from a Dietitian

While bone broth is excellent, its collagen content can vary widely. I recommend making your own from grass-fed bones, simmering for at least eight to twenty-four hours to maximize collagen extraction. Here's my personal favorite strategy: Buy a whole chicken with the skin on from a local farmer and make a chicken soup at least once a month, consuming both the broth and the skin as medicine. This traditional practice delivers more than just collagen—it provides a full spectrum of nutrients in their most bioavailable form.

For my busy clients who can't regularly make bone broth, I suggest a two-pronged approach: Combine supplemental collagen (specifically look for types I and III) with natural whole-food collagen sources: fish with skin, chicken skin, and pig's skin. These traditional foods, often overlooked in modern nutrition, are actually potent sources of natural collagen that your body recognizes and uses efficiently.

Protein for Easy Weight Loss

Let me tell you about Liza, a client who came to me from California. She was proud of her strict vegan juice cleanse lifestyle but frustrated with constant cravings and stubborn excess weight. Despite consuming mountains of leafy greens and plant protein, she felt hungry all the time and couldn't understand why her body wasn't cooperating with her wellness goals.

During our first session, her eyes filled with tears as she admitted to dreaming about steak. Yes, literally dreaming about it. Her body was desperately trying to tell her something, but she was too caught up in her clean-eating ideology to listen. After reviewing her labs, I noticed classic signs of protein deficiency: low iron, depleted B_{12}, and hormonal imbalances.

Here's what I told her: "Let's use animal protein as medicine." We started small—introducing wild-caught fish and organic eggs during her luteal and menstrual phase when her body needed it most. Eventually, we added grass-fed meat once a month, treating it with the respect of a therapeutic intervention rather than a dietary failure.

The transformation was remarkable. Within three months, her cravings vanished, her energy soared, and she finally started losing weight. But here's the really interesting part: By spacing her protein intake throughout the day (20 to 40 g per meal), her body started functioning like a well-oiled machine.

The science behind this is fascinating: Protein isn't just about muscles. It's the building block for every hormone in your body, crucial for immune function and essential for metabolic health. When you don't get enough, your body literally starts breaking down its own tissue to access the amino acids it desperately needs.

Pro Tip from a Dietitian

Think of protein timing like feeding a fire. You wouldn't dump all your firewood on at once and expect it to burn efficiently all day. Instead, space your protein intake evenly:

- **Breakfast:** 20–40 g (e.g., pasture-raised eggs with quinoa or a protein-rich smoothie with hemp seeds)
- **Lunch:** 20–40 g (e.g., wild-caught salmon, sardines, or lentil salad with tahini)
- **Dinner:** 20–40 g (e.g., organic chicken, tofu stir-fry, or bean and veggie chili)

Liza now follows this protocol while maintaining her love for plant foods. She's found her balance—mostly plant-based but with strategic animal protein when her body signals the need. She's not just surviving; she's thriving.

Prioritize variety in your protein sources. Incorporate a mix of high-quality animal- and plant-based proteins into your meals to get a wide spectrum of nutrients. Spread your protein intake evenly across meals, aiming for 30 to 40 g per meal, and consider adding collagen or bone broth to your diet for additional gut and skin benefits. Remember, muscle isn't just about aesthetics—it's your longevity insurance. By fueling your body with the right proteins, you're giving it the tools to thrive at every stage of life.

Eat protein at every meal, but make sure it's a ***complete*** protein. Animal products tend to have the highest amount of the most bioavailable proteins, followed by legumes (beans), whole grains (rice, wheat, corn), and root vegetables such as sweet potatoes, carrots, beets, parsnips, and turnips. Animal protein (from meat, eggs, fish, and milk) contains all the essential amino acids our bodies need and are normally referred to as "complete" or "high biological value" protein. Protein derived from plants lacks one or two essential amino acids. However, a good combination of plant-based protein can be of equal value to animal protein. For example, legumes lack methionine but have adequate amounts of lysine. Whole grains, on the one hand, lack lysine but have a lot of methionine. Therefore, a mixture of rice and beans will supply all the essential amino acids—which is why so many different cultures have cuisines that pair the two.

Why Your Body Craves Fats

Fat is one of the body's most fundamental building blocks. The trillions of cells that make up our bodies rely on high-quality fats to maintain their membranes, produce hormones, and power mitochondria—critical for brain function, metabolism, and overall energy. These dietary fats go beyond being a mere source of fuel; they act as essential signaling molecules that regulate numerous processes in the body. From enhancing nutrient absorption and maintaining cellular integrity to supporting sustainable weight management, healthy fats are vital for optimal functioning and longevity.

Let me tell you about Sharon, a twenty-seven-year-old who came to my office terrified of fats. She'd meticulously cut every bit of fat from her diet, proudly choosing egg whites over whole eggs and dry salads over anything with olive oil. Despite her ultra-low-fat diet, she couldn't lose those last ten pounds, and she struggled with constant hunger, dry skin, and brain fog.

When I ran her gut-health test, the results were eye-opening. Her microbiome showed a severe deficiency in short-chain fatty acids—those crucial compounds that feed your gut lining and support your metabolism. Without adequate healthy fats, her mitochondria (those tiny powerhouses in your cells) were struggling to produce energy.

Most people don't realize that healthy fats aren't just calories—they're cellular communication tools. Your brain is 60 percent fat. Your hormones need fat to function. Your mitochondria prefer fat as a clean energy source. When you deprive your body of healthy fats, you're essentially shutting down your internal communication system.

I started Sharon on what I call the healthy foodie protocol (see recipes in Chapter 9):

- **Morning:** 1 tablespoon medium-chain triglycerides (MCT) oil in her coffee
- **Breakfast:** Whole eggs with ¼ avocado
- **Lunch:** Salads dressed with olive oil and apple cider vinegar
- **Dinner:** Wild-caught fatty fish rich in omega-3s

- **Snacks:** Raw macadamia nuts or a handful of sunflower seeds

Her transformation was remarkable. Within weeks, her skin developed a healthy glow, her mind became sharper, her energy stabilized throughout the day, she started losing weight naturally—and most surprisingly, her constant hunger and frequent cravings, especially for sweet treats, began to fade.

Omega-3 Fatty Acids: Delicious Sources for Every Lifestyle

As a dietitian who loves good food, I believe healthy eating should always be delicious and satisfying. Omega-3 fatty acids, essential for brain health, heart health, and reducing inflammation, are a perfect example of how nutrient-dense foods can also be enjoyable. Whether you love seafood or prefer plant-based options, there's an omega-3-rich food for your particular plate and palate.

The Three Forms of Omega-3s

Alpha-linolenic acid (ALA) is found primarily in plant sources like flax seeds, chia seeds, and walnuts. While beneficial, ALA needs to be converted by your body into eicosapentaenoic acid (EPA) and docosahexaenoic acid (DHA)—a process that isn't very efficient in humans, with conversion rates typically below 5 percent.

EPA and DHA are the more bioavailable forms, found predominantly in fatty fish like salmon, mackerel, and sardines. DHA is particularly crucial for brain health and development, while EPA plays a significant role in reducing inflammation. Think of DHA as your brain's building block and EPA as your body's inflammation manager.

I often recommend that my clients focus on getting EPA and DHA directly from cold-water fatty fish or high-quality fish oil supplements while using plant-based ALA sources as a complement rather than their primary omega-3 source. For vegetarians and vegans, I suggest algae-based supplements, as algae is where fish originally get their EPA and DHA.

Best-Tasting Omega-3 Sources of Seafood (EPA and DHA)

- **Salmon.** Grill it, bake it, or enjoy it smoked—salmon is a flavorful powerhouse of omega-3s. Pair it with a bright citrus glaze or a side of roasted vegetables for a satisfying meal.
- **Sardines.** Packed with flavor, sardines are perfect on whole-grain toast or tossed into a vibrant pasta dish.
- **Mackerel and anchovies.** Add these to salads, pizzas, or spreads for a savory omega-3 boost.
- **Trout.** A milder fish that's perfect for grilling with herbs or baking with a squeeze of lemon.

Plant-Based Omega-3s (ALA)

- **Flaxseeds.** Sprinkle ground flaxseeds into smoothies, oatmeal, or homemade energy bars for a nutty flavor and a nutrient-packed punch.
- **Chia seeds.** Soak them in almond milk for a creamy pudding, mix into smoothies, or use as a crunchy topping.
- **Walnuts.** Add to salads or baked goods, or snack on them roasted for a simple, heart-healthy treat.
- **Hemp seeds.** Perfect for sprinkling over avocado toast, soups, or smoothie bowls for a subtle, nutty taste.

How to Maximize Omega-3s from Plants

Plant-based omega-3s (ALA) offer great versatility, but converting ALA into EPA and DHA—the active forms our bodies need—is inefficient. To bridge this gap, I recommend incorporating into your routine algae oil, a vegan-friendly source of EPA and DHA. It's a simple way to enjoy all the health benefits of omega-3s without sacrificing your plant-based preferences.

For those relying on plant sources, balance your diet with foods that enhance omega-3 conversion, like zinc-rich nuts, seeds, and legumes, or vitamin B_6–packed options like sweet potatoes and bananas.

As someone who enjoys good food, I often combine seafood and plant-based sources for variety. A grilled salmon fillet with a side of quinoa topped with hemp seeds, or a vibrant salad with walnuts and a drizzle of chia seed vinaigrette, is both nourishing and delicious. The beauty of omega-3-rich foods is that they're as versatile as they are healthy. Whether you're indulging in a Mediterranean-inspired seafood dinner or sprinkling superfoods into your morning smoothie, there's a way to make omega-3s a flavorful part of your day. In the final chapter, I share a few of my favorite Mediterranean cuisine–inspired recipes with anchovies! After all, eating well isn't just about health—it's about enjoying the process.

Quality Versus Quantity

Think of healthy fats like the oil you put in a luxury car—you wouldn't put cheap gas in a Ferrari, right? The same goes for your body. Here's my quality hierarchy for fats (organic only):

- **Avocados (Hass variety).** Serving size matters! For standard Hass avocados (not the larger Florida type), the general guideline is:

    Women: ¼ of a medium Hass avocado per serving

    Men: ½ of a medium Hass avocado per serving

- **Extra virgin olive oil.** Choose cold pressed from small farms, 1 to 2 tablespoons per meal.

- **Cold-pressed coconut oil:** 1 tablespoon per serving
- **Raw nuts and seeds:** 1 to 2 tablespoons per serving

The Golden Elixir: Why I Prescribe Ghee

I specifically recommend ghee for its unique molecular structure and therapeutic properties. Through the clarification process at 485°F (252°C), all milk solids are removed, leaving behind a pure butterfat rich in fat-soluble vitamins A, D, E, and K_2, along with butyric acid—a short-chain fatty acid that studies show directly nourishes colonocytes (cells lining the colon) and reduces intestinal inflammation. The removal of proteins casein and lactose makes ghee suitable for most dairy-sensitive individuals, while its high smoke point of 485°F makes it optimal for high-heat cooking without producing harmful oxidative compounds.

Pro Tip from a Dietitian

For optimal therapeutic benefits, I recommend 1 teaspoon of ghee per meal, not exceeding 3 to 4 tablespoons weekly. This dosage provides approximately 1.5 to 2 grams of butyrate daily—the amount shown in clinical studies to support gut barrier function and reduce inflammatory markers. Always choose organic, grass-fed ghee to ensure maximum concentrations of conjugated linoleic acid (CLA) and vitamin K_2, both crucial for metabolic health and proper calcium utilization.

The Fat Fear Factor: A Science-Based Perspective

Let's address misconceptions about dietary fats and cholesterol. The connection between dietary fat and heart disease is far more nuanced than we once thought. Research from the Harvard School of Public Health demonstrates that plaque formation is more closely linked to inflammation and oxidative stress than to dietary cholesterol alone. Your liver produces about 80 percent of your body's cholesterol, but its ability to process and balance LDL (often called bad cholesterol) depends heavily on your overall dietary pattern. *The key lies in supporting your liver's natural detoxification pathways while maintaining healthy cholesterol metabolism.*

This is why I teach my clients *the art of balance rather than restriction.* Enjoying that grass-fed steak or butter isn't the problem—the issue arises when we don't provide our body with the tools it needs for proper cholesterol metabolism. Fiber acts as your liver's best friend, binding to excess cholesterol and facilitating its removal through natural detoxification pathways. Think of fiber as your body's internal cleaning crew, helping to maintain cholesterol balance without deprivation.

Pro Tip from a Dietitian

Structure your plate this way: Fill half with colorful, fiber-rich plants, a quarter with quality animal protein (no need to choose only lean cuts), and the remaining quarter with complex carbohydrates. This ratio provides the perfect balance of nutrients to support healthy cholesterol metabolism while nourishing your body with the fats it needs for optimal function.

Here's the fascinating truth: Cholesterol is so essential for human life that every cell membrane in your body contains it. Your brain is 60 percent fat, and cholesterol serves as a crucial building block for hormone production. The issue isn't about avoiding cholesterol. It's about supporting your body's natural ability to process and utilize it effectively. Think about it now. What will you order next time to complement your steak? My recommendation: Add broccoli, spinach, and mushrooms, and consider starting with a vegetarian appetizer like a soup or a salad. No need to shy away from animal protein; balance is key.

The Truth About Dairy Fats

The low-fat dairy trend, born from misguided fears about cholesterol in the 1980s, led to a generation of fat-phobic consumers reaching for skim milk and fat-free yogurt. From a functional medicine perspective, I see daily the metabolic consequences of this shift. Research now demonstrates that full-fat dairy consumption is actually associated with lower risks of metabolic syndrome and improved insulin sensitivity, likely due to the unique fatty acid profile and fat-soluble nutrients that are stripped away in fat-free versions. Here the issue of quality arises. That's why I highly recommend choosing dairy from local farmers who raise their animals humanely and avoid excessive antibiotics or chemically treated feed. If that's not accessible or within budget, look for certified organic, grass-fed dairy at your local grocery store, the next best alternative for quality and purity.

For clients with dairy sensitivity, I specifically recommend fermented products from goat and sheep milk sources. These alternatives contain different protein structures—primarily A2 beta-casein versus the A1 found in cow's milk—making them significantly less inflammatory for most people. Clinical studies show that caprine (goat) and ovine (sheep) dairy products contain higher levels of MCTs, conjugated linoleic acid, and uniquely structured proteins that enhance mineral absorption. Additionally, their naturally smaller fat globules make them easier to digest.

The Science of Smart Carbohydrates

In my career as a dietitian, I've witnessed every diet trend, including seeing carbohydrates transform from dietary staple to public enemy number one. The truth is both more complex and simpler than the headlines suggest. Let me break down the science of why not all carbohydrates are created equal and how to find the right carbohydrates that love you back.

Historically, traditional cultures thrived on complex carbohydrates—from Japanese centenarians with their sweet potatoes to Mediterranean communities with their ancient grains. The problem isn't carbohydrates; it's the modern mutation of what we call "carbs." Let's get specific.

Damaging carbohydrates:

- Processed white flour products that spike blood sugar and create inflammation
- High-fructose corn syrup that overwhelms liver function
- Ultraprocessed snack foods stripped of fiber and nutrients
- Sugary beverages that deliver pure glucose without any nutritional benefit

Nourishing carbohydrates:

- Root vegetables rich in resistant starch that feeds beneficial gut bacteria
- Ancient grains containing prebiotic fibers that support microbiome diversity
- Legumes offering slow-release energy and protective compounds
- Fresh fruits packed with polyphenols and fiber

The difference lies in how these carbohydrates affect your blood sugar, gut bacteria, and cellular health. Modern research from the American Gut Project shows that people consuming at least thirty different plant species weekly have the most robust microbiomes—and many of these plants are complex carbohydrates.

Let me break this down into what I call the carb hierarchy.

Nonstarchy vegetables. Think of broccoli, kale, and Brussels sprouts as premium fuel for your gut bacteria. These vegetables contain unique fiber compounds called **glucosinolates** that not only feed beneficial bacteria but also support your body's natural detoxification pathways. People who eat a wide variety of plant foods—rich in different fibers and polyphenols—tend to have higher levels of short-chain fatty acid–producing bacteria like *Faecalibacterium prausnitzii*, which are linked to reduced inflammation, improved gut lining integrity, and stronger immune function.

Starchy vegetables. Sweet potatoes, winter squash, and beets aren't just delicious—they're packed with resistant starch that acts as a prebiotic, feeding the beneficial bacteria in your gut. These complex carbohydrates release glucose slowly, providing sustained energy without the blood-sugar roller coaster of refined carbs.

Ancient grains. Quinoa, millet, and traditional oats contain **beta-glucans**—powerful fiber compounds that can reduce inflammation and strengthen your gut barrier. These grains create SCFAs that literally feed the cells lining your intestines when broken down by your gut bacteria.

Pro Tip from a Dietitian

Incorporate quinoa, oats, sweet potatoes, purple potatoes, beans, or buckwheat into your meals for sustained energy, but consume in moderation: only one to two servings per day.

Opt for whole-grain-sprouted bread or quinoa in small portions alongside your veggies and protein for balanced meals. Different-colored potatoes offer varying amounts of antioxidants. For instance, purple sweet potatoes that are purple both on the outside and inside—such as the Okinawan or Stokes Purple varieties—are especially high in anthocyanins, potent antioxidants linked to brain and heart health. However, some sweet potatoes may have purple skin but white flesh, such as the Japanese sweet potato *(Satsumaimo)*. These still offer fiber and complex carbs but contain less anthocyanin than their fully purple counterparts. When shopping, check the label or variety name, and look for Stokes Purple if you're specifically seeking the antioxidant benefits of deep-purple flesh.

The Good Food: Enjoying Real Food Without Guilt

Food is more than fuel—it's connection, joy, and culture. As a dietitian and a foodie, I encourage my clients to embrace real foods they love, even those considered indulgent, with a mindful and balanced approach to nutrition and longevity science in mind.

Let me simplify the often-confusing concept of whole foods with a straightforward truth: If you can't recognize what's in it, it's not a whole food. When you look at a piece of wild-caught salmon, an avocado, or a sweet potato, you know exactly what you're getting. No ingredient label needed. No surprises.

I love explaining this to my clients using real-world examples. Compare a chicken breast to a "vegan chicken nugget." Chicken breast is one ingredient. The vegan nugget? I recently counted seventeen different ingredients, including methylcellulose and isolated soy proteins. Sure, it's marketed with a health halo, but your body knows the difference.

Take the "impossibly delicious" plant-based burger that's all the rage. Created in a lab with processed soy, artificial flavorings, and numerous additives, it's a far cry from the simple, nutrient-dense whole foods your body recognizes and knows how to process. A grass-fed beef burger, in contrast, is just that: beef, with all its natural nutrients intact.

This is why I encourage even my busiest clients to try cooking, even if just a few days a week. Making a simple meal helps you understand how real food comes together. When you sauté fresh vegetables in olive oil or grill a piece of fish, you see exactly what goes into your meal. There's no mystery, no hidden ingredients, no preservatives or artificial anything.

My recommendation is to make whole foods 80 percent of your diet—think ripe tomatoes from the farmers' market or grown in your backyard, perfectly roasted sweet potatoes, fresh berries, raw nuts, grass-fed meats, and wild-caught fish—because your body has evolved over thousands of years to recognize, digest, and use these natural foods in ways that no food scientist in a lab, no matter how clever, can improve upon or replicate.

Fiber and Protein at Every Meal Makes Staying Slim and Strong No Big Deal

Take steak, for example. A palm-size portion paired with roasted vegetables isn't just a delicious meal—it's a perfect example of how traditional foods can support our health when properly balanced.

While the steak provides protein, iron, and essential nutrients, the fiber-rich vegetables alongside it are doing crucial behind-the-scenes work.

That crusty sourdough bread with butter you love? It's not the villain it's been made out to be—especially when you choose whole-grain or traditionally fermented sourdough paired with high-quality butter, such as grass-fed options like Kerrygold, which are rich in omega-3s and fat-soluble vitamins. The real issue isn't that these foods are inherently bad—it's that we often don't support our liver's daily processing of LDL and HDL cholesterol with enough fiber.

Remember the 80/20 rule? It's your ticket to both health and pleasure. When you eat whole, clean foods 80 percent of the time, those luxury indulgences not only become more special—they can actually contribute to your nutrition goals. Take uni (sea urchin), foie gras, and oysters—these aren't just decadent treats; they're nutrient powerhouses when enjoyed in moderation.

Fiber: Your Gut's Best Friend and Beauty Secret

Let me tell you why I'm obsessed with fiber—eating it is a nonnegotiable—and why it should be on your plate at every meal. Fiber from green leafy vegetables acts as your gut's internal cleansing crew, adding bulk, supporting regularity, and helping sweep out toxins and excess cholesterol. The result? A healthier microbiome and that natural, energized glow from the inside out.

Here's what fascinates me as a dietitian: Fiber isn't just mechanical bulk—it's premium food for your beneficial gut bacteria. When you feed these good guys fiber-rich foods, they multiply and flourish, naturally crowding out the troublemakers in your gut. This is why I can't emphasize enough the importance of getting fiber at every meal, and it's easier than you might think.

Now, let's talk about your daily nutritional champions: fiber-rich foods, especially those green leafy vegetables. In the nutrition world, we call these "free foods" for good reason. They're so low in calories yet so high in nutrients that you can eat them in unlimited amounts. Want to know the secret to sustainable health? At every meal, fill half your plate with these nutritional superstars.

Pro Tip from a Dietitian

Think about feeding your gut bacteria like tending a garden. Different beneficial bacteria thrive on different types of fiber. Aim for at least five to seven different-colored plants per day and thirty-plus different plants per week to support a diverse microbiome. Your gut bacteria will thank you with better mood and energy, and a more active metabolism.

Anti-Inflammatory Foods That Would Benefit Everyone

In my approach as a food-loving dietitian, I tend to focus on nutrient-dense foods that bring the best bang for your buck—meaning lots of goodness and health benefits packed into each calorie. Everyone should know about these superheroes and incorporate them into their daily life.

Let me share what I've learned from years of helping clients optimize their nutrition while maintaining their love for food. These aren't just random superfoods. They're powerful allies that can transform your health without sacrificing pleasure.

Here are the five foundational foods for an anti-inflammatory diet that I covered during my TEDx Talk "How to Fall in Love with the Food That Loves You Back."

1. **Leafy greens.** Rich in antioxidants, kale, spinach, and arugula support detoxification and reduce inflammation.
2. **Berries.** Berries like blueberries, raspberries, blackberries, strawberries, cranberries, and acai are rich in anthocyanins and polyphenols, powerful antioxidants that help combat oxidative stress, reduce inflammation, and support a diverse and resilient gut microbiome.
3. **Fatty fish.** SMASH fish—salmon, mackerel, anchovies, sardines, and herring—are excellent sources of omega-3 fatty acids (EPA and DHA). These healthy fats are essential for reducing systemic inflammation and promoting brain and gut health. They also support the gut lining and improve microbial balance.
4. **Spices and herbs.** Spices and herbs do more than add flavor—they're functional medicine.
   - **Turmeric,** rich in *curcumin*, helps reduce inflammation and supports gut lining integrity.
   - **Ginger** aids digestion and reduces nausea and bloating.
   - **Cinnamon** helps stabilize blood sugar and has antimicrobial effects.
   - **Oregano, thyme, rosemary, and basil** have antioxidant, antimicrobial, and anti-inflammatory properties.
   - **Cilantro and parsley** support detoxification pathways and liver health.
5. **Fermented foods.** Sauerkraut, kimchi, and yogurt introduce beneficial bacteria into your gut, enhancing digestion and immunity.

Let's look at these in more detail because these foods definitely love you back!

Optimize Omega-3 Intake

Prioritize foods rich in omega-3 fats two to four times per week. These include wild-caught Alaskan seafood such as Vital Choice's wild-caught salmon, sardines, mackerel, and anchovies. Wild-caught seafood is high in anti-inflammatory omega-3 fats, which promote brain and heart health.

I'm passionate about wild-caught seafood, particularly when it comes to fatty fish like salmon, because the difference between wild caught and farm raised isn't just about sustainability. It's about nutrient density and cellular health.

Look at the color difference: Wild salmon displays a deep, vibrant orange-red hue while farm raised often appears pale pink. This isn't just aesthetics—it's a visible marker of astaxanthin content, a powerful antioxidant responsible for that rich coloring. Wild salmon contains up to 400 percent more astaxanthin than farm raised because these fish naturally consume astaxanthin-rich krill and algae in their native environment. Farm-raised salmon, by contrast, often get their color from compounds added to their feed.

To support inflammation balance and brain health, I recommend incorporating wild-caught Alaskan seafood—like salmon, sardines, mackerel, and anchovies—into your meals, a few times per week, as a reliable source of omega-3s. Here's why: Wild fish not only provide those essential anti-inflammatory omega-3 fats for brain and heart health, they also come with significantly lower levels of contaminants. Farm-raised fish are often exposed to antibiotics, pesticides, and higher levels of polychlorinated biphenyls due to their confined environment and artificial feed. Farm-raised salmon contains persistent organic pollutants, added red dye for color, higher saturated fats, and antibiotics from their feed.

Pro Tip from a Dietitian

When shopping for salmon, use the color test—that bright orange-red hue isn't just Instagram-worthy, it's a reliable indicator of higher astaxanthin content and wild origin. Sustainability guidelines are also available through organizations like the NOAA and the Marine Stewardship Council that can help you make informed seafood choices. This applies to all types of seafood—wild-caught shrimp, lobster, and crab typically have more vibrant coloring and better nutritional profiles than their farm-raised counterparts. Grill or bake fish with olive oil, lemon, and herbs for a simple, nutrient-packed meal.

Include fatty fish in your diet two to four times a week to get optimal levels of EPA and DHA. If you're not eating fatty fish at least two to four times per week, you may not be getting enough EPA and DHA, the essential omega-3 fatty acids. In that case, consider supplementing with a high-quality fish oil or algae oil to support brain, heart, and inflammatory health.

Cruciferous Vegetables Daily: Your Liver's Best Friend

What fascinates me about cruciferous vegetables, and why do I discuss them with all my clients concerned about detoxification and cellular health? These green powerhouses contain a unique compound called glucoraphanin that converts to sulforaphane—a potent activator of our body's natural detoxification pathways. As a dietitian focused on functional medicine, I specifically recommend these vegetables for their ability to support both Phase I and Phase II liver detoxification processes.

Research from Johns Hopkins Univcrsity shows that sulforaphane activates the NRF2 pathway—your body's master regulator of antioxidant response. This activation triggers over two hundred protective genes and detoxification enzymes. Most fascinating is how *broccoli sprouts contain up to one hundred times more sulforaphane potential than mature broccoli.*

Here's my clinical protocol for maximizing these benefits: Chop your cruciferous vegetables (broccoli, Brussels sprouts, cauliflower, or kale) and let them rest for forty-five minutes before cooking. This waiting period is crucial—it allows the enzyme myrosinase to convert glucoraphanin into active sulforaphane. When cooking, I recommend light steaming or quick sautéing to preserve these beneficial compounds. The goal is one cup daily, divided between meals to maintain steady detoxification support.

Pro Tip from a Dietitian

Adding mustard to cooked cruciferous vegetables, like broccoli or Brussels sprouts, can significantly boost their health benefits. Mustard contains the enzyme myrosinase, which helps convert glucosinolates in cruciferous vegetables into sulforaphane, a potent compound known for its anti-inflammatory and cancer-fighting properties. This simple pairing enhances the bioavailability of sulforaphane, maximizing the vegetables' protective effects.

For those who can't tolerate the taste of cruciferous vegetables, microgreens and sprouts offer concentrated nutrition in a smaller package. Just one ounce of broccoli sprouts provides the sulforaphane equivalent of nearly two pounds of mature broccoli.

Antioxidants: Your Cellular Shields

Antioxidants and polyphenols are remarkably beneficial for your health and work at the cellular level. These compounds aren't just nutrients—they're your body's natural defense system against oxidative damage and premature aging. Here's the science of why these colorful compounds are crucial for optimal health.

Think of antioxidants as your cellular bodyguards. Flavonoids, polyphenols, and specific vitamins give fruits and berries their deep, rich colors, and here's the key principle I share with my clients: *The deeper the color, the higher the antioxidant content*. If it can stain your clothes, it's probably exceptional for your cells!

Pro Tip from a Dietitian

Timing matters with antioxidants. I recommend consuming berries on an empty stomach or with protein for optimal absorption and never with iron supplements as they can interfere with absorption.

Water-soluble antioxidants clear from your system within hours, which is why daily consumption is crucial. I recommend one half to one cup of berries daily, prioritizing wild varieties, which research shows contain up to ten times more antioxidants than cultivated ones. Wild blueberries, pomegranates, tart cherries, and cranberries top my list for their exceptional polyphenol content and proven benefits for brain health and DNA protection.

For optimal cellular protection, I guide my clients to combine different sources: dark chocolate (at least 70 percent cacao) for its unique flavanols, green tea for its EGCG (epigallocatechin gallate) content, and extra virgin olive oil for its hydroxytyrosol—a polyphenol so powerful the European Food Safety Authority issued a health claim for its protection against LDL oxidation.

Spices and Herbs: Ancient Medicine in Your Kitchen

Longevity studies from *National Geographic*'s Blue Zones research reveal a fascinating pattern: Populations living beyond one hundred years consistently incorporate specific herbs and spices into their daily diet. These aren't just flavor enhancers—they're potent medicinal compounds used in small amounts but with remarkable consistency.

These powerful medicinal allies include the following:

- **Turmeric and ginger.** Not just digestion supporters, research shows they actively promote healthy gut motility and reduce inflammation. I guide clients to combine these in a golden latte with plant-based milk and a pinch of black pepper to enhance absorption by 2,000 percent.
- **Garlic.** Rich in quercetin, a flavonoid that studies show enhances immune cell function. One daily clove provides significant antimicrobial and cardiovascular benefits.
- **Oregano.** Contains potent antimicrobial and antiparasitic compounds. Traditional Greek usage—sprinkling it fresh on salads—maximizes its active compounds.
- **Parsley, cilantro, thyme, rosemary.** These Mediterranean staples contain unique polyphenols that support detoxification pathways. Fresh application, as practiced in Greece, preserves their volatile beneficial compounds.
- **Clove and cinnamon.** Beyond their warming properties, these spices demonstrate remarkable blood sugar–regulating

effects. Just ¼ teaspoon of cinnamon on your morning yogurt, oatmeal, or sliced apple can help stabilize glucose levels.

Fermented Foods That Love Your Gut

I've seen so many transformations in my clients who incorporate fermented foods into their daily routine. These living foods aren't just condiments—they're powerful tools for gut health and immune system modulation. The science behind why these ancient foods are more relevant than ever is fascinating.

Recent groundbreaking research from Stanford University demonstrates that a diet rich in fermented foods increases microbiome diversity and reduces inflammatory markers more effectively than even a high-fiber diet. What particularly excites me is how these foods deliver not just probiotics but also postbiotics—metabolites produced during fermentation that directly support gut barrier function and immune regulation. Here's my clinical protocol for incorporating these powerful foods:

Start with small amounts—think 1 tablespoon of raw sauerkraut with meals, gradually increasing to ¼ cup daily. Traditional ferments like kimchi, properly fermented pickles (explained below), and plain kefir contain diverse strains of beneficial bacteria that you simply can't get from a supplement. Each fermented food offers unique benefits: Kimchi provides *Lactobacillus plantarum* essential for gut barrier function, while kefir contains up to fifty different microorganisms that support immune function and mental health through the gut-brain axis.

Pro Tip from a Dietitian

It is very easy to prepare homemade sauerkraut, kimchi, or pickles—and yes, I include a simple recipe in the next section to help you get started. Look for another recipe in Chapter 9. However, if you are pinched for time, here is what to seek out in store-bought products.

When shopping, check the ingredient list: True ferments should contain only vegetables, salt, and maybe spices, never vinegar or preservatives. Look for truly fermented products in the refrigerated section—they should be unpasteurized to retain live cultures. Don't be fooled by shelf-stable pickles and sauerkraut sitting at room temperature in grocery store aisles; these products typically contain vinegar rather than undergoing true fermentation, meaning they lack the beneficial live bacteria we're seeking. That naturally tangy, sour taste in properly fermented foods isn't just flavor—it's a sign of active beneficial compounds working for your health.

Hydration for Cellular Health

Do not miss your chance to get an extra load of nutrients and vitamins from hydration for cellular nourishment. Here's the science behind specific drinks I recommend to my clients for maximum health benefits with minimal sugar impact.

- **Green matcha tea** stands out for its unique catechin EGCG, shown in clinical studies to enhance cognitive function and support cellular autophagy. Unlike steeped green tea, matcha provides the whole leaf's nutrients, delivering 137 times more antioxidants than regular green tea.
- **Tart cherry juice** is a powerful tool for uric acid balance and inflammation reduction that I've been recommending since my dietetic residency years when we were prescribing tart cherry pills for those with gout. Research demonstrates its

ability to reduce postexercise muscle damage and improve sleep quality through its natural melatonin content. However, I specifically recommend diluting it 1:3 with water to maintain its benefits while avoiding glucose spikes.

- **Pomegranate juice,** particularly organic varieties in glass bottles, has shown remarkable effects on memory and cognitive function. Studies reveal its punicalagins can cross the blood-brain barrier, potentially protecting against neurodegenerative conditions. Again, I recommend a 1:3 dilution to optimize antioxidant benefits while managing sugar content.

Pro Tip from a Dietitian

For store-bought kombucha and coconut water, check sugar content carefully; many brands contain as much sugar as soda— up to 15 g per bottle, which is more than 3 teaspoons of sugar! (Natural, yes, but still sugar!) I guide my clients to dilute these drinks 1:1 with water or choose low-sugar varieties, aiming to keep total sugar under 4 g per serving.

Caffeine: Benefits and How to Drink

I see wide variations in caffeine sensitivity among my clients. While research confirms coffee's and green tea's impressive antioxidant benefits for Parkinson's disease and type 2 diabetes prevention, timing and method of consumption matter significantly. I always teach my clients to *avoid caffeine on an empty stomach*. This isn't just old wisdom, it's supported by research showing that consuming caffeine without food can increase cortisol levels by up to 30 percent and potentially damage the stomach's mucosal lining.

Instead, I guide my clients to consume their coffee or matcha with a balanced meal containing protein, healthy fats, and fiber. This combination creates a time-release effect, allowing for steady caffeine absorption while protecting the digestive system. For example, have your morning coffee with eggs, avocado, and lox, or enjoy matcha as part of a balanced lunch with salad and protein.

Pro Tip from a Dietitian

Originally, milk was added to coffee to balance its acidity and because milk is a complete food containing proteins, fats, and carbohydrates. Nowadays, when a lot of people are avoiding cow's milk, the best substitution is actually soy milk because of its high protein and fat content, along with its comprehensive nutrient profile. However, because in America soybeans have a very bad reputation due to GMO quality, I often recommend choosing either organic soy milk or macadamia and hemp milk to add to a cup of coffee.

Dietitian's Guide to Nutrient Density: Nature's Superheroes

I've explored countless "superfoods," but let me share what I consider true nutritional royalty. These aren't trendy marketing gimmicks. They're foods backed both by ancestral wisdom and modern science. Even if you're not ready to incorporate them today, understanding their benefits is crucial for your health journey.

1. The Ultimate Multivitamin: Organ Meats

Let me start with what I consider nature's most potent multivitamin: beef liver. When I tell my clients about liver's nutrient profile, they're often skeptical until they see the numbers: Just one 4-ounce serving provides 731 percent of your daily vitamin A, 988 percent of vitamin B_{12}, and more bioavailable iron than any plant source.

The beauty of organ meats extends beyond liver. Traditional cultures understood the wisdom of nose-to-tail eating—from *trippa alla roma* (Roman-style beef stomach) to delicacies like sweetbreads (the thymus or pancreas glands typically of calves or lambs) and beef tongue. These cuts aren't just sustainable; they're nutrient powerhouses with unique compound profiles you won't find in muscle meat. Take heart, for example: It's the best food source of CoQ10, crucial for cellular energy production.

Pro Tip from a Dietitian

For organ meat newcomers, start with just one ounce of grass-fed liver weekly. I often recommend freezing it in small portions and adding it to ground beef dishes where its flavor is less noticeable. If you're not ready for whole organ meats, desiccated liver capsules from quality sources can provide similar benefits.

2. Antioxidant Powerhouses: Cranberries, Seabuckthorn, Goji, Elderberry

Cranberries deserve special attention for their unique proanthocyanidins (PACs), which prevent bacterial adhesion in the urinary tract—a mechanism not found in any other berry. With only 4 grams of sugar per cup, compared to 15 grams in blueberries, they offer potent antioxidants without the glycemic impact. I make fresh cranberry sauce at Thanksgiving (with fruit, not sugar), but outside the holidays, cranberries can be hard to find fresh due to seasonality.

That's why I recommend buying them frozen during the offseason or stocking up on fresh cranberries when available and freezing them yourself to toss into smoothies year-round.

In my practice, I recommend cranberries regularly during flu season for their immune-boosting vitamin C content, and I've seen recurring UTI symptoms resolve within weeks of daily cranberry intake.

Elderberry has scientifically validated antiviral properties. Clinical studies show it can reduce flu duration by four days through its specific antiviral compounds, sambucol and anthocyanins. I recommend it to my clients in powdered form to be added to smoothies, especially to those who travel and socialize a lot, or at the first sign of illness—300 mg of standardized extract, four times daily.

Pro Tip from a Dietitian

Add a handful of fresh or frozen unsweetened cranberries to your salads, smoothies, or salad dressings. You can also blend frozen cranberries into your smoothies for a tart, refreshing twist on traditional blueberry smoothies and delicious easy-to-make elderberry gummies—recipes in Chapter 9!

3. Phospholipid Omega-3 for Brain Health: Red Caviar

Red caviar isn't just a luxury. It's a therapeutic food, what I call "nature's supplement capsule," containing phospholipid-bound omega-3s that cross the blood-brain barrier 100 percent more effectively than fish oil. Just 1 tablespoon provides 2 g of these highly bioavailable fatty acids, plus astaxanthin for added antioxidant protection. Most fascinating is its choline content—1 ounce of red caviar provides 100 percent of your daily requirement for this crucial brain nutrient.

Pro Tip from a Dietitian

For optimal absorption, consume red caviar with a source of fat like avocado and scrambled eggs. I recommend 1 to 2 tablespoons three times weekly, particularly during periods of high cognitive demand or stress. Store it properly in the refrigerator at the coldest setting for maximum preservation of its delicate nutrients.

4. Nature's Zinc Dynamo for Healthy Skin from Within: Oysters

Oysters deliver more zinc per serving than any other food—just 3 ounces provide 673 percent of your daily zinc requirement. Zinc activates over three hundred enzymes in the body and plays a key role in thyroid function, immune support, skin barrier repair, and gut lining integrity. I've seen clients with recurring skin issues or acne experience noticeable improvements within weeks of adding oysters to their diet.

While raw oysters are popular, they do carry a higher risk of bacterial contamination, especially for individuals with compromised immunity. If you're concerned, you can absolutely enjoy them cooked, such as steamed, grilled, or baked. For optimal nutrient content, I recommend choosing the freshest oysters available, ideally locally sourced or regionally imported, to retain both flavor and health benefits. In addition to zinc, oysters are also rich in vitamin D, B_{12}, and selenium, making them a nutrient-dense food for overall health and vitality.

Clinical research shows that oysters' unique zinc-copper ratio (8:1) makes them effective for immune system modulation and testosterone production. They also contain unique marine peptides that support collagen synthesis more effectively than supplements.

Pro Tip from a Dietitian

Consume oysters at least once a month—up to three times per month, ideally aligned with moon cycles—as they are one of the most concentrated natural sources of zinc, selenium, copper, and B_{12}, all essential for thyroid health, immune function, and hormone balance. When you're ordering oysters at a bar or restaurant, always ask how fresh they are—and don't hesitate to smell them before eating. Fresh oysters should smell like the ocean, not fishy. Always choose sustainably sourced options and consume them within twenty-four hours of shucking for both safety and optimal flavor. Enjoy them raw with a squeeze of lemon or vinegar, and add them to seafood stews and chowders for a nutrient-packed meal.

5. Daily Liver Detox with Mustard Greens

Mustard greens are part of the cruciferous vegetable family, containing specific glucosinolates that trigger phase 2 liver detoxification more effectively than other cruciferous vegetables. Their unique compound, sinigrin, converts to allyl isothiocyanate—shown to increase detox enzyme production.

The bitter compounds in these greens stimulate bile production, digestive enzymes, and cholecystokinin hormone release, improving fat digestion and vitamin and nutrient absorption. When my clients learn to incorporate these greens three times weekly, we often see improved liver enzymes within three months. Bitter greens like arugula, radicchio, dandelion greens, endive, escarole, frisée, watercress, chicory, mustard greens, rapini, kale, turnip greens, beet greens, collard greens, and Swiss chard are nutrient dense and support digestion with their bold, distinctive flavors.

Pro Tip from a Dietitian

Massage mustard greens with olive oil and let sit for ten minutes before cooking to maximize nutrient availability. Add dandelion, endive, watercress, or mustard greens to your salads and stir-fries, or blend them into a Green Goddess Smoothie (recipe in Chapter 9). For a delicious side dish, sauté mustard greens with garlic and olive oil, or mix them into soups and stews for an extra nutrient boost.

6. The Perfect Healthy Fat: Avocado

Avocados aren't only healthy fat—they're brain architecture. Their specific ratio of oleic acid to alpha-linolenic acid (13:1) perfectly matches our brain cell membrane composition. One medium avocado provides 4.5 g of fiber and 250 mg of glutathione—our body's master antioxidant.

Avocados are a fantastic source of heart-healthy monounsaturated fats, which support hormone balance, brain function, and cardiovascular health. They're also rich in fiber, potassium, and antioxidants like lutein and zeaxanthin, which is beneficial for eye health. Most fascinating is their impact on lutein (carotenoid antioxidant) absorption. Studies show that adding half an avocado to a meal increases carotenoid absorption by 400 percent and improves cognitive function scores in adults over age sixty. The healthy fats in avocados help you absorb fat-soluble vitamins (A, D, E, and K) from other foods, making them a perfect addition to any meal.

> ### *Pro Tip from a Dietitian*
>
> For optimal nutrient absorption, consume ¼ of an avocado with each meal containing fat-soluble vitamins. Store unripe avocados in a paper bag with a banana to speed up ripening naturally. Add ¼ to ½ of an avocado to your morning smoothie, slice it on top of salads, or mash it as a spread for toast. Pair it with a source of protein like eggs or salmon for a balanced meal.

7. From Forest Floor to Medicine Cabinet: Mushrooms

In eastern Russia when I was growing up, mushroom foraging was more than just gathering food—it was a meditative ritual passed down through generations on how to connect with nature to find these little hidden gems under the leaves. I remember early-morning walks with my grandparents in the woods, basket in hand, learning to identify different species. This ancestral wisdom sparked my fascination with mushrooms' therapeutic properties, which modern science now validates through extensive research.

What most people don't realize is that mushrooms are nutritional powerhouses, containing all nine essential amino acids in a highly bioavailable form. Their protein content ranges from 20 to 30 percent by dry weight, making them one of the few complete protein sources in the plant kingdom. This is why I specifically recommend them to my vegetarian clients who need to diversify their protein sources beyond legumes and grains.

Reishi, which I now sip as an evening tea just as my grandmother taught me, has been shown to contain specific beta-glucans that enhance natural killer cell activity by up to 300 percent. Clinical studies demonstrate that its triterpenes help regulate sleep cycles and reduce cortisol levels.

Lion's mane holds a special place in my clinical recommendations for cognitive support. Its unique compounds, hericenones and erinacines, stimulate nerve growth factor production, supporting brain plasticity and repair. I've seen remarkable improvements in my clients' mental clarity within eight to twelve weeks of consistent use.

Turkey tail, perhaps the most researched medicinal mushroom, contains polysaccharide-K, clinically proven to enhance immune system function. Its diversity of prebiotic compounds supports microbiome health in ways that synthetic probiotics cannot match.

Pro Tip from a Dietitian

For optimal absorption of mushrooms' beneficial compounds, always heat them. The cell walls contain chitin, which needs thermal processing to release bioactive compounds. When making mushroom tea, gently simmer (don't boil) for at least twenty minutes, and add a small amount of healthy fat like coconut oil to enhance absorption of fat-soluble compounds.

8. Nature's Eternal Medicine: Honey

Did you know that honey is the only food that never goes bad? Honey was discovered in ancient Egyptian tombs still perfectly preserved after thousands of years. This eternal shelf life comes from its unique biochemical properties: a precise combination of low moisture content, high acidity, and naturally occurring hydrogen peroxide that creates an environment where no bacteria can survive.

I recommend honey as a functional food for its therapeutic applications. Manuka honey, with its unique methylglyoxal compound, demonstrates antibacterial potency that can be precisely measured through its unique manuka factor (UMF) rating. Clinical studies show that Manuka honey that is rated UMF 15+ can effectively combat antibiotic-resistant bacteria and support wound healing.

Here's my protocol for diabetic clients who want to benefit from honey's medicinal properties without blood sugar spikes: Always pair it with protein and fat sources. For example, combine 1 teaspoon of honey with 1 tablespoon of almond butter, or dilute it in warm water with 1 teaspoon of coconut oil. This combination slows glucose absorption while still providing honey's antibacterial and anti-inflammatory benefits.

Pro Tip from a Dietitian

Look for raw, unfiltered honey that crystallizes naturally, indicating the presence of beneficial compounds and the absence of processing. For therapeutic use, I recommend taking 1 teaspoon of Manuka honey (UMF 15+ or higher) mixed with warm (not hot) water first thing in the morning, at least twenty minutes before breakfast.

Your Journey to Nutrient-Rich Living

We've explored nature's most powerful foods—from the depths of the ocean with mineral-rich oysters to the ancient wisdom of medicinal mushrooms. Each of these foods carries its own unique symphony of compounds that support your body's intricate systems. But this is just the beginning of your journey into optimal nutrition.

Key Takeaways

- **Quality matters more than quantity.** Choose organic, grass-fed, and wild-caught sources whenever possible. Use the Environmental Working Group's annual Clean Fifteen and Dirty Dozen lists as your shopping guide. These resources show which conventional produce is safe to consume (like avocados, sweet corn, and pineapples) and which are heavily pesticide-treated and worth buying organic (such as strawberries, spinach, and kale). This practical approach helps you invest in organic options where it matters most.
- **Nutrient density is your secret weapon.** Focus on foods that deliver maximum benefits per calorie.
- **Timing is crucial.** *When* you eat is often as important as what you eat.
- **Food synergy works.** Combine foods strategically to enhance nutrient absorption.
- **Listen to your body.** What works for others may not work for you.
- **Balance is key.** The 80/20 rule allows for both optimal nutrition and life's pleasures.

In Chapter 8, "Feed Your Hunger for Health," I dive deeper into advanced nutrients and longevity compounds that can take your health to the next level. You'll learn how to strategically use these nutrients to support healthy aging and vitality.

But knowing what to eat is only half the equation. In our next chapter, I'll show you how to transform this knowledge into sustainable daily habits. Because let's be real—life doesn't always happen in your perfectly stocked kitchen. Whether you're traveling for business, dining out with friends, or juggling a busy schedule, you need strategies that work in the real world.

I'll share my tried-and-true methods for incorporating these nutrient-dense foods into your lifestyle in ways that are both practical and enjoyable. Because remember—*this isn't about perfection, it's about progress and joy on your path to optimal health.*

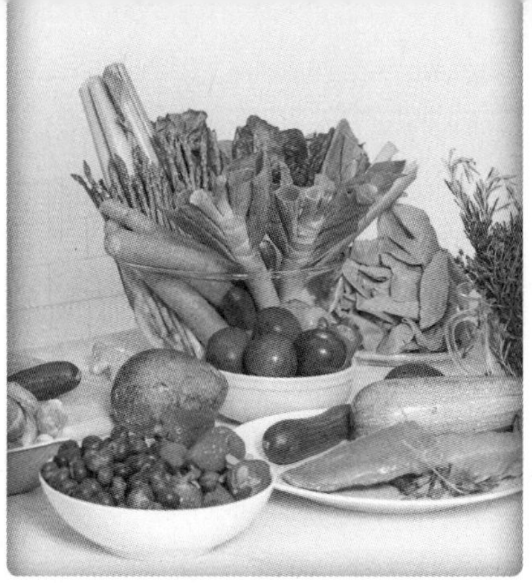

Chapter 6

Food Rules for Living Life to the Fullest: Dining Out, at Home, and While Traveling

Love: The Secret Ingredient for Longevity

One vital ingredient going beyond nutrients and calories that I recommend adding to every meal is love. As a dietitian who understands both the science and soul of nutrition, I've seen how our emotional connection to food transforms not just what we eat but how our bodies process it.

Bring sexy back in the kitchen! This isn't just a catchy phrase—it's about restoring the loving relationship between you and your optimal nourishment. When you approach food preparation and eating with joy and intention, you're creating a sustainable healthy lifestyle that can be passed on to future generations. Love isn't just an emotion here; it's literally the energy of life and a key to longevity.

Beyond counting macros or following rigid rules, the most successful clients in my practice are those who've learned to infuse their nutrition journey with love, joy, and pleasure. They make weekly farmers' market visits a whole family adventure—taking their kids to farms to explore, play with animals (and get exposure to different microbes that build a child's immunity!), and buy local produce for the week. By focusing on nutrient-dense, high-quality foods, you create an approach that supports your busy lifestyle without feeling restricted.

This isn't about perfection. It's about treating your hardworking self with the nourishment you deserve. When you choose foods that make you resilient and help you glow from within, you're not just eating; you're investing in your ability to achieve all your ambitious dreams in a more fulfilling way.

When we cook with love, a certain alchemy happens, an almost mystical transformation. The food somehow tastes better. It's more nourishing! We feel it in our bones. We just can't get enough, but at the same time, we feel deeply satiated. We've all experienced this, the amazing feeling of eating Mom's or Grandma's home-cooked food—whether it's chicken soup or spaghetti with meatballs—prepared with love, intention, and care.

Eating with love is a pillar of the Foodie Diet. It's a love of food that is balanced with a love for ourselves, our bodies, and our families. Focus on restoring the loving relationship between you and your food for optimal nourishment and a sustainably healthier lifestyle that you can pass on to the next generation. I truly believe that love is the secret elixir, the energy of life—which means that it is the key to longevity! Science has proven in countless different ways that people with more love in their lives live longer and healthier. Functional medicine expert Dr. Mark Hyman explains, "When we have a deep connection with someone, it literally changes our gene expression"—a powerful reminder of how relationships can influence our biology. Inversely, conflicted relationships make us more susceptible to increased inflammation, disease, and accelerated aging.

The healing power of food prepared with love isn't just a nice idea. There's real science behind it. Research by Dr. Masaru Emoto, author of *The Hidden Messages in Water*, suggests that positive thoughts and words can influence the molecular structure of water, forming more coherent, symmetrical crystal patterns. As he wrote, "Water reflects the consciousness of the human mind." When you cook with love, your emotions are absorbed by the food. Anyone who eats it can feel the love that went into it and be nourished by that love.

When you feed yourself healthy food, do it from a place of loving care. Ask your body, *What nutrients do you want and need right now?* Ask yourself, *How can I treat myself with nourishing food? What can I put in my body that will make me more resilient, that will help me glow from within, and support me to achieve my dreams in a healthier, more fulfilling way?*

For me, cooking is the ultimate act of self-love and self-respect. It is taking responsibility for what I put in my body and the intentions and energy with which it is made. As a busy New Yorker, my life changed when I started to view cooking, not just manicures and massages, as an act of self-care. This turned food preparation from a chore into a daily ritual. Bringing more mindfulness to the process of buying and prepping food, getting creative with the process, and cooking with kind and loving intentions is truly game-changing.

As foodies, we want to *cook with love and eat with mindfulness.* That means slowing down to truly experience and savor what's on our plate, using all five of our senses. Mindful eating increases awareness, pleasure, digestion, absorption, and metabolic action. Notice how your food looks, feels, and tastes in your mouth. The color. The scent. The texture. How do the smell and thought of your meal make you feel? Savoring your meal is an act of gratitude to your body and the earth that created your food. You can take it a step further by recognizing where your food came from and all the labor involved in getting it from the soil to your plate.

Breathwork to Improve Digestion

My favorite way to eat with greater awareness—and incidentally to improve digestive function—is to take three deep breaths before eating. This is by far one of the best and most efficient ways to improve digestion; it helps your body switch into a parasympathetic nervous system, responsible for rest-and-digest mode, for your body to prioritize digestion. Try this little breathwork practice before dinner tonight to help you directly experience the gut-brain connection and stimulate the vagus nerve:

> Close your eyes to bring your full attention inward. Place your hands on your heart and feel its steady rhythm. Take a deep breath in, then exhale slowly. Breathe in again, and this time, let your exhale stretch even longer, releasing tension with each out-breath. Once more, take a deep inhale, followed by an even slower exhale. As you breathe out, notice your heart rate slowing. This calming rhythm signals

your brain that it's safe to rest, digest, and thrive. You might even feel a slight increase in saliva production—your body's natural readiness to absorb nutrients. With this moment of mindfulness, you are now prepared to eat with gratitude and intention.

Here are some strategies and hacks for incorporating more mindfulness into your meals:

- **Stop multitasking.** When we eat unconsciously, we eat more. Avoid multitasking while eating. Eat while you eat—nothing more! Turn off the phone, TV, email, and computer, and take a break from media while you focus on nourishing yourself.
- **Avoid stressful conversations.** During meals, the body should be in a rest-and-digest state, not in fight-or-flight mode, which disrupts digestion by diverting blood flow away from the stomach. There's a Russian saying taught to children, "When I eat, I am deaf and mute," emphasizing that meals are not the time for emotional or stressful discussions. Many of my high-performing clients conduct much of their business over dinner, often while multitasking or under pressure—leading to frequent indigestion and weight gain. Interestingly, some trace this pattern back to childhood meals that were less about nourishment and more about problem-solving, discipline, or stress-filled conversations, setting the stage for a lifelong association between eating and tension.

These conversations can lead to cortisol spikes, which divert blood flow away from the digestive tract, thereby suppressing digestion and leading to GI issues, poor sleep, and increased fat storage. This physiological response can result in symptoms such as bloating, abdominal discomfort, and nutrient malabsorption. I recommend avoiding emotional topics during meals and waiting at least thirty to sixty minutes afterward before discussing anything potentially stressful to give your body time to focus on properly digesting and absorbing nutrients.

- **Remember the twenty-minute rule.** Every meal should take at least twenty minutes. By eating consciously and slowly, you allow yourself to honor your true hunger and satiety needs by providing ample time for your brain to get the signal that your stomach is full.
- **"Take five" before your meal.** In less than a minute, boost your metabolism and shift your nervous system into rest-and-digest mode: Breathe in through your nose for a count of five, pause briefly, and exhale through your mouth for a count of five. Repeat this cycle five times or until you feel fully relaxed and present. Placing a hand on your belly encourages deeper, diaphragmatic breathing, which enhances your connection to the moment and your meal. While three breaths can center you in a pinch, dedicating a full minute or adding a gratitude prayer deepens the experience and allows you to fully appreciate the nourishment before you. This mindfulness practice not only optimizes digestion with enzymatic sufficiency but also transforms the act of eating into a grounding and nourishing ritual. Trust me, the world is not going to fall apart if you disconnect from it for twenty-five minutes and focus fully on your meal three times a day.
- **Offer gratitude and a blessing.** Here is my favorite prayer for expressing thanks before your meal. This simple yet profound prayer is something I share with my clients, inspired by my yoga teachings and the mindfulness practices of my role model, Gisele Bündchen. Watching how she instills this

awareness in her children reminds me to honor the interconnectedness of life and the nourishment we receive from nature.

- **A prayer of gratitude for food.** Take a moment to pause and appreciate the food before you. Reflect on the journey it took to reach your plate, acknowledging everyone who contributed to its presence. From the farmers who nurtured and cared for the produce to the workers who gathered, packaged, and delivered it to the stores or farmers' markets, every step is a labor of love and effort. Consider the hands that picked and prepared this food—those who shopped for it, washed it, and cooked it—all to nourish you. This food will soon become part of you, providing life and energy.

With love and mindfulness, every meal becomes an opportunity to care for yourself and others.

Dear food,

I offer thanks to the farmers who nurtured the soil and tended the plants with care.

I give gratitude for the harvesters, packagers, and transporters who made it possible for this nourishment to arrive in my hands.

I bless the people who stocked it on the shelves, the ones who selected it with love, and those who prepared and served it—whether that's a family member, a chef, or myself.

I acknowledge the sacred cycle of life and effort that brought this meal to my plate.

May this food nourish my body, calm my mind, and open my heart.

With mindfulness, I receive it with love and gratitude.

Enjoy every bite! Fun fact: You may notice that you need less food to feel satiated when you are fully present at each bite focusing on flavor, texture, and taste. Take a moment to pause and truly appreciate the food before you. Reflect on the journey it took to reach your plate.

Food blessing. When you sit down, hover your hands above the plate and take three deep breaths, connecting with and feeling gratitude for what you're about to eat. Sense the energy exchange with your food, offering a blessing to each meal while being intentional and present in the moment. Forgive yourself for times when you've eaten on the go—distracted and without thought. Pausing before you begin to eat provides a moment of deep gratitude and quiet reflection, helping you feel more connected and conscientious about what you're choosing to put in your body. This small practice can heighten your awareness of the nutrients you consume that fuel and nourish you, keeping you healthy and strong. Food is a gift—a gift you give yourself to function at your best—so blessing your meal reinforces that purpose and intention.

The Science Behind Mindful Eating

Every bite you take has the power to boost your hormones, and your metabolic and mental health for longevity when consumed mindfully. Here's the science behind it:

Neuroscience of mindful eating. Mindful eating involves being fully present during meals, which enhances digestion and nutrient absorption. Studies have shown that focusing on the flavors, textures, and smells of food activates the prefrontal cortex, responsible for self-control and decision-making, helping regulate eating behaviors and preventing overeating.

Hormones and the gut-brain connection. As we discussed in Chapter 4, the gut produces about 90 percent of the body's serotonin, a neurotransmitter that regulates mood. Nutrient-dense foods, like salmon and flaxseeds rich in omega-3 fatty acids, reduce inflammation and support brain health. Dark chocolate increases endorphin levels, enhancing mood. Fermented foods like yogurt and kimchi supply probiotics that maintain a healthy gut microbiome, essential for serotonin synthesis. A balanced gut microbiome also influences the production of GABA, a neurotransmitter that promotes relaxation and reduces anxiety.

Research on happiness. A diet rich in fruits, vegetables, and whole foods is linked to higher levels of happiness and well-being. Antioxidants in fruits and vegetables reduce oxidative stress, associated with mood disorders. Foods high in tryptophan, such as turkey and bananas, boost serotonin levels, promoting a sense of well-being. Omega-3 fatty acids have been shown to reduce symptoms of depression and anxiety, enhancing overall happiness.

Healthy weight and longevity. Mindful eating supports maintaining a healthy weight. By paying attention to hunger and satiety cues, individuals are less likely to overeat. A study in the journal *Obesity Reviews* found that mindful eating interventions led to significant weight loss and improved eating behaviors. Maintaining a healthy weight is crucial for longevity, as obesity is linked to chronic diseases like diabetes, cardiovascular disease, and certain cancers.

Nutrient-rich foods and longevity. Eating a variety of fruits and vegetables provides essential vitamins and minerals that energize and uplift mood. Leafy greens, berries, and nuts are packed with nutrients that boost energy and improve mental clarity. Research in the *Journal of Nutrition* shows that plant-based diets are associated with a lower risk of mortality and increased lifespan. Nutrients like fiber, antioxidants, and phytochemicals in these foods contribute to long-term health and longevity.

Mindful eating isn't just about food choices; it's about how you eat. Savoring meals without distractions allows you to connect with your body's needs, leading to better overall health and happiness. By eating mindfully, you harness the power of nutrition to support your mental and physical well-being. Every bite becomes a step toward a healthier, happier, and longer life. *Remember, food is medicine, and changing your attitude toward food may change your relationship with life!*

How to Eat What You Want Without Sabotaging Your Health

Through trial and error, I've learned some marvelous hacks for protecting my long-term health while occasionally indulging in some of my favorite foods.

Rescue Remedy for Sweet Tooth

As I've shared, I'm genetically predisposed to diabetes, so it's important that I'm mindful of my sugar and carbohydrate consumption. I know what happens when I eat too much sugar: It spikes my insulin, and then I feel like crap when it crashes back down. Just the other day, I ate too many of my favorite cookies, these special crunchy wafers that you can only find in European markets. I'm a sucker for them. I totally overdid it, but I didn't sweat it. There's an herbal blend I love called Blood Sugar Breakthrough, which is available online through BiOptimizers.com and select health retailers, which I use for my clients who are working on weight loss and metabolism. It's a selection of herbs that stabilize your insulin levels (banana leaf extract, cinnamon, etc.) and promote healthy blood-sugar levels. I popped a few of those, took a moment to let go of any guilt, recommitted to loving my body, and went back to my day. I recommend taking it shortly before or right after eating sugar-spiking foods to help support healthy glucose and insulin responses.

I recommend supplements and products containing proven ingredients to help my clients balance their blood sugar effectively, especially during holidays when many people struggle to avoid temptations. Ingredients like berberine, which improves insulin sensitivity and reduces glucose production, and chromium picolinate, which enhances glucose metabolism, are key components for glycemic control. Alpha-lipoic acid (ALA) acts as a potent antioxidant, improving insulin sensitivity and reducing oxidative stress, while magnesium supports insulin signaling and glucose metabolism. Soluble fibers such as psyllium or glucomannan stabilize postmeal blood sugar by slowing carbohydrate absorption, and cinnamon extract helps reduce fasting glucose and postprandial spikes. Additionally, fenugreek and gymnema sylvestre aid in glucose regulation by slowing absorption and supporting insulin secretion while also reducing sugar cravings. Zinc is critical for insulin production and action, and bitter melon provides compounds that mimic insulin, enhancing glucose uptake. Together, these ingredients offer a science-backed approach to blood-sugar management, and I often recommend tailored blends that combine their synergistic benefits to meet individual needs.

Balance It Out with a Breakfast Salad

I am famous for my breakfast salads. If you overeat one night, I recommend skipping breakfast the next morning or making a colorful, nutritious breakfast salad (you'll find the formula in "A Foodie's Lunch, How to Master Any Salad" in Chapter 9). You just grab a big bowl and throw in some mixed greens, tomato, radishes, carrots, endive, and whatever veggies you have on hand, plus a poached, pan-fried, or hard-boiled egg (if you can tolerate eggs). Trust me, your body will *love* it. It's gonna feel so darn good to eat this after a night of pizza or splurging on dessert. You might just get addicted to starting the day with a light and nutrient-dense bowl of veggies because it feels and tastes so amazing!

Alcohol Detox and Balancing Strategies

Balancing alcohol intake and supporting the body's detoxification processes can be achieved through a combination of natural remedies, food choices, and advanced supplements.

- Hydration is essential for flushing ethanol. Choosing to enjoy a glass of wine or a cocktail on occasion is no big deal—but if you do, drink a glass of water with your drink, follow each alcoholic beverage with 8 to 12 ounces of water, and add electrolytes to your water if you have more than two drinks.
- Activated charcoal at bedtime and also in the morning are good ways to support your liver in removing toxins. Charcoal binds to toxins in your digestive system, helping to reduce their absorption and aiding your liver in detoxification. Always drink plenty of water alongside charcoal to stay hydrated and enhance its effectiveness in flushing out toxins.

- Supplements like milk thistle, known for its hepatoprotective properties, turmeric for its anti-inflammatory benefits, and dandelion root for liver support enhance the body's natural detox capabilities.
- Key nutrients such as B vitamins, which are depleted by alcohol, L-glutamine to support gut health, and vitamin C as an antioxidant play a huge role in recovery.

Hangover Recovery Recommendations

If you find yourself nursing a hangover, combine the previous recommendations with the following strategies to help your body recover and restore balance:

- Start your day with green juices made from cucumber, celery, leafy greens, and spices. These are rich in hydration and antioxidants, providing essential nutrients to combat inflammation and oxidative stress. Pair your juice with probiotic-rich foods like pickled beets or kimchi, along with protein-packed eggs, to restore gut health and support liver detoxification.
- Hydration is key. Drink plenty of water or electrolyte-rich beverages like unsweetened coconut water or clean electrolyte formulas such as LMNT (no sugar, no artificial colors), Nuun Sport (clean version), or Re-Lyte by Redmond, which offer essential minerals without added sugars or synthetic ingredients. These formulas contain essential electrolytes like sodium, potassium, and magnesium, which are crucial for replenishing what is lost during alcohol metabolism. Incorporate potassium-rich foods such as bananas, avocados, and sweet potatoes to further restore electrolyte balance and prevent junk-food cravings.

- Antioxidants like vitamin C from citrus fruits and glutathione precursors from eggs neutralize free radicals, protecting your cells from damage. To ease nausea, sip on ginger-lemon tea, and for headaches or muscle tension, include magnesium-rich foods like pistachio nuts and pumpkin seeds in your meal.
- Advanced detox strategies include NAD+ supplementation or medically supervised IV therapy, which support cellular repair and can help reduce withdrawal symptoms.
- Incorporating regular exercise, quality sleep, and sauna therapy further promotes the body's natural detox processes for faster recovery and long-term health.

Personalized Nutrition

I recently designed a diet plan for one of my clients, a French athlete living in Paris who loved to eat out at the city's incredible restaurants. When I diagnosed him with gluten and dairy intolerance after extensive testing, he was so excited that he'd found the key to finally feeling better after years of digestive discomfort and persistent brain fog. "That's it!" he said. "No more gluten and no more dairy. Easy."

I loved the enthusiasm, but let's be real: Challenges lie ahead too. He might start out with good willpower while his friends enjoyed beautiful cheese plates and bowls of tagliatelle, but eventually he was likely to cave. So I gave him my go-to dining-out rules to use that 80-plus percent of the time he wanted to stay on track with the foods he knew his body loved. But I also gave him all the necessary buffers and safety nets to use if he ended up indulging (either mindfully or just in a moment of weakness), including these:

- Digestive enzymes containing dipeptidyl peptidase IV (DPP-IV) and aspergillopepsin (ASP), an enzyme derived from *Aspergillus niger*, have been found to work synergistically with DPP-IV to break down gluten proteins more efficiently than either enzyme alone can help break down gluten proteins, reducing adverse reactions.

- Probiotics, particularly strains like *Lactobacillus plantarum* and *Lactobacillus paracasei*, have been shown to enhance gluten digestion and support gut health.
- Additionally, L-glutamine supplementation aids in repairing the intestinal lining for better gut integrity. It's important to note that while these supplements can support digestive health, they are not substitutes for a gluten-free diet.

This athlete now had everything he needed to stick to his protocol on most occasions while still enjoying the culinary good life—an omakase dinner, a beautifully grilled branzino, or hanger steak. But he also had a damage-control plan to help manage a lapse—no guilt, just simple tools to minimize the damage and get quickly back on track.

I want you to enjoy life and eat what you love. We've all seen photos of beautiful, thin models chowing down on pizza. That's the purpose of this chapter: to teach you how to be the one eating pizza or crème brûlée or drinking champagne while still feeling great and staying completely loyal to your health goals. You can be that person who says honestly, "I eat everything." You just have to follow two simple rules when it comes to the foods that you love but your body doesn't:

1. You eat them very rarely. It's a special occasion. You mindfully indulge when it's really worth it, but you don't overdo it.
2. When you do overindulge—and we all do; that's what holidays and celebrations are for!—you counterbalance any

negative effects with some simple damage-control measures and get back on track with the foods that make your body run right.

This is what the Foodie Diet is all about: *Eat what you want, but do it right.*

I use this client as an example because this is such a common scenario. So many people are gluten- and dairy-intolerant but still want to enjoy eating out, which is why I'll share my rules for how to eat out healthfully and all my hacks for managing the crisis. For gluten, for example, there are the specific enzymes I recommended to my clients that are designed to ease discomfort and minimize the ill effects of consuming delicious wheat-containing baked products (and they really work). And my list of herbs, supplements, enzymes, and detox hacks to use after you indulge (or *over*indulge) to create more balance with other common trigger foods like dairy, sugar, and alcohol. A moment of mindful indulgence (or caving to your cravings) doesn't have to derail you.

When You Overindulge

When you've overindulged during a celebration or enjoyed a particularly heavy meal at Carbone (an Italian classic restaurant notoriously famous for very rich and heavy classical dishes), use these targeted herbs, supplements, enzymes, and detox hacks to support digestion and recovery.

Herbs

- **Ginger.** Brew fresh ginger tea by steeping a few slices of peeled ginger root in hot water for ten minutes. Add a squeeze of lemon juice to support detoxification and enhance antioxidant activity. Fresh ginger is generally more potent than many store-bought ginger tea products, which may contain lower concentrations of active compounds. Ginger helps reduce bloating, stimulates gastric emptying, and eases nausea.

- **Peppermint.** Brewed from loose leaves or a high-quality tea bag, peppermint can help relax the digestive tract and relieve gas, bloating, and cramping. For more targeted relief, peppermint oil capsules offer a more concentrated form and are often used in clinical digestive protocols.
- **Fennel seeds.** Chew a teaspoon of fennel seeds after meals to support digestion and reduce bloating. Fennel seeds contain volatile oils that relax intestinal muscles, ease gas buildup, and stimulate bile flow for smoother digestion. They're a traditional remedy in many cultures and are especially helpful after heavier meals.

Supplements

- **Probiotics.** Take a high-potency multistrain probiotic supplement to restore gut flora and reduce inflammation after a heavy meal. Strains like *Lactobacillus acidophilus and Bifidobacterium longum* are particularly effective.
- **Magnesium citrate.** Use magnesium to relieve bloating and constipation. A dose of 200 to 400 mg in the evening can help relax the digestive tract and promote regular bowel movements. However, for some people, it may increase the urge to go to the bathroom, so consider starting with a lower dose or taking it earlier in the evening to avoid sleep disruptions.
- **Milk thistle.** This herb supports liver detoxification and aids in breaking down alcohol or fatty foods. Look for a supplement with silymarin for maximum benefit.

Enzymes

- **Digestive enzyme blends.** Look for formulas containing lipase, protease, and amylase to break down fats, proteins, and carbohydrates. For best results, take one dose with your largest meal—or with each meal, if needed—based on your symptoms and practitioner guidance.
- **Betaine HCl with pepsin.** If you struggle with low stomach acid, this supplement enhances protein digestion and reduces postmeal discomfort.
- **DPP-IV enzymes.** Specifically helpful if you consumed gluten, these enzymes help break down gluten peptides to ease digestive strain.

Detox Hacks

- **Activated charcoal.** Take 500 to 1,000 mg after your meal to bind toxins and reduce bloating. Avoid taking it with other supplements to prevent interference with absorption.
- **Apple cider vinegar.** Dilute 1 to 2 tablespoons in a glass of water and drink before or after your meal to aid digestion and balance blood sugar levels.
- **Herbal teas.** Dandelion tea promotes liver detoxification, while fennel tea reduces gas and bloating. Chamomile tea can help relax the stomach and ease discomfort.
- **Walking.** A ten- to fifteen-minute walk after eating can aid digestion and prevent food from sitting in your stomach. This light activity supports better blood sugar balance, gastric motility, and reduces bloating.

By incorporating these specific recommendations, you can quickly support your digestive system, alleviate discomfort, and return to feeling your best after overindulging. Don't be too hard on yourself—it happens to the best of us!

Dining Out

It's important to find a diet that suits your unique body and goals. Experiment with the balance of macronutrients—alcohol, carbohydrates, protein, and fats—to determine what works best for you.

For the majority of the time, when you're committed to eating healthy while eating out, it's all about *mindful preparation.* I always say: Don't be a victim to the menu!

I would never suggest you forgo the fun of dining out while gathering with friends and family or traveling. These are some of my go-to guidelines to help you succeed while dining out.

Be Graciously Obnoxious!

Be clear about your needs, and do not accept any food that does not nourish or support you. Do not assume that you're being impolite; you are simply taking care of yourself assertively. Not only is this not rude, but you may even inspire someone else to have more clarity and fortitude around committing to their own self-care needs.

Don't Be Afraid to Ask Questions

Before dining out, it's helpful to research the restaurant online to learn about their sourcing practices. If the menu still lacks transparency, don't hesitate to ask your server. Many are trained to answer questions about where ingredients come from, especially when it comes to **seasonal, local, or sustainable options.** If they don't know, that information is useful in itself.

Questions to Ask

- "Is the fish on the menu wild caught or farm raised? Is it a fresh, local catch?"
- "Where is your beef sourced from? Could I have it simply grilled, please?"

- "Are your vegetables locally sourced? Could you prepare them Mediterranean-style with olive oil and garlic, using less oil?"

Asking questions helps you make informed choices and signals to the restaurant that customers value transparency and quality.

Call the shots. When you can, be the one to choose the restaurant. I often recommend going with Mediterranean or Greek cuisine when possible, as this will likely give you the widest range of healthy options without having to limit yourself to a vegan or vegetarian restaurant.

Ask for water. Drink one to two glasses of spring water before your meal to reduce your appetite (it really works!). Just make sure it's room temperature, as ice-cold water can slow down your digestion. However, I recommend avoiding water during and right after meals. Here's why: Drinking too much liquid with food dilutes your stomach acid and digestive enzymes, potentially compromising nutrient absorption and slowing down the breakdown of proteins. I tell my clients to wait at least thirty minutes after eating before drinking water again, giving their bodies time to properly digest and absorb nutrients from their meal.

I recommend choosing still spring water whenever possible, as it's typically lower in additives than sparkling varieties. If true spring water isn't available, the next best option is filtered water from a high-quality home filtration system. When dining out, opt for still water as well—sparkling water, while refreshing, contains carbon dioxide, which can cause bloating or discomfort in some individuals, especially when consumed alongside a meal. Additionally, the natural minerals found in still spring water support electrolyte balance and overall hydration without the potential gastric irritation that carbonation might cause. Opting for still spring water ensures a gentle and restorative hydration experience, complementing the nourishment of the meal without unnecessary digestive strain.

Ask for a simple preparation (and beware of sauces). Grilled fish with an entire plate of steamed vegetables with some olive oil and lemon drizzled on top is a delicious, satisfying, and nutrient-filled option. Be cautious with store-bought sauces, dressings, and dips as they're often laden with hidden sugars, inflammatory oils, gluten, or low-quality dairy. However, Mediterranean staples like tzatziki, hummus, and tahini-based dips can be great options when made from whole ingredients—or better yet, homemade.

Follow "hari hachi bu." Do as the Okinawans do and stop eating when you are 80 percent full. Instead of eating until you are *full*, eat until you are *no longer hungry*! Don't hesitate to bring leftovers home—even too much of the right foods may spike insulin levels.

How to Order

Look on the side-dish menu, such as for vegetable selections, for your anti-inflammatory foods. This is a great way to start your meal. I recommend ordering green leafy or colorful nonstarchy vegetables for starters (like peppers, Brussels sprouts, or mushrooms), as well as more vegetables to complement the main course, such as carrots or baked potato.

When you know what to look for, you can easily ask the server for it without even looking at the menu: "What green vegetables can you recommend, simply cooked, sauteed or grilled?" Here's how to make the most of your vegetable options at different types of restaurants.

Greek Restaurants: Embrace the Greens

Greek cuisine is a treasure trove of nutrient-dense vegetables, so take advantage of it!

- **Horta (boiled dandelion greens).** This traditional dish is often overlooked, but it's a powerhouse for your liver. Dandelion greens support natural detoxification, helping your body cleanse and rejuvenate. Pair them with a drizzle of olive oil and a squeeze of lemon for a refreshing, liver-loving side dish.
- **Mountain herbal tea.** Don't miss out on the unique herbal teas often offered at Greek restaurants. Ask for *tsai tou vounou* (mountain tea), a potent herbal brew made from wild plants that are rich in antioxidants and known to stimulate digestive enzymes—perfect for aiding digestion after your meal!

Asian Restaurants: Go Green with Flavor

Asian cuisine offers an array of delicious, vegetable-centric dishes. Here's what to look for:

- **Bok choy.** This leafy green is a staple in Asian cuisine, but it's often sautéed with too much oil. Be sure to ask for it prepared with less oil to keep it light and healthy. Bok choy is loaded with vitamins A, C, and K, and its high water content makes it a great hydrating side.
- **Watercress salad.** Watercress is not just a garnish! This peppery green is rich in antioxidants and supports liver health. Order it as an appetizer to get your greens in early and set the tone for a balanced meal.

Italian Restaurants: Leafy Delights for Detox

Italian restaurants may be known for pasta and pizza, but they also have fantastic vegetable offerings that are often found in the side-dish section:

- **Arugula salad.** Arugula is a detox dynamo, often included as a side or in salads. It's high in chlorophyll, which helps cleanse the liver and supports overall detoxification. Look for it as a side dish or as the base of a salad with some lemon and shaved Parmesan.

- **Radicchio and insalata tricolore.** These salads typically feature a mix of bitter greens like radicchio, arugula, and endive. The bitterness is fantastic for stimulating digestive enzymes and supporting liver function. Enjoy this combo to balance out a richer main course.

Planning Ahead for Eating Out

A little planning can make all the difference when dining out, allowing you to enjoy your meal while avoiding the guilt of making last-minute decisions without considering nutritional value. The reason certain cuisines (Italian, for example!) are so exceptional is their reliance on a minimal number of ingredients, elevated by the quality of those ingredients and the care in preparation. This is why it's essential to spend some time researching restaurants where the chef is deeply committed to sourcing high-quality ingredients and preparing them with skill and intention. By choosing places that prioritize food quality, you ensure that your dining experience is enjoyable *and* aligned with your health goals!

Look for Restaurants That List the Source of Their Ingredients

A great indicator of a restaurant's commitment to quality is when they proudly name the farms or locations their ingredients come from. Whether it's Colorado lamb, California avocados, or grass-fed beef from a local ranch, restaurants that specify the origin of their ingredients are usually more committed to quality and transparency. They're not just serving food; they're telling a story about it.

I get very excited when I notice these details and make sure to ask the manager questions about the farm. They are usually eager to share the background, especially regarding seasonal produce and nutrient density, which depends on soil health, farming practices, and the harvest's timing. Seasonal ingredients are often at their peak in both flavor and nutritional value, as they are grown and harvested in alignment with nature's rhythms. Understanding the effort that goes into ensuring these factors makes it even more rewarding to appreciate what is proudly presented to the consumer. My goal is to teach you how to recognize and value this dedication.

How to Spot Food Sources on the Menu

- Look for phrases like "sourced from [farm name]," "Colorado-raised lamb," or "locally grown in [region]."
- Some menus even list the specific farms or fisheries, like "Sustainable salmon from Skuna Bay" or "Heritage pork from Niman Ranch."

Knowing where your food comes from ensures it's fresh, sustainably sourced, and often of higher nutritional quality. These restaurants typically avoid mass-produced cheap ingredients and opt for seasonal, local, and ethically sourced ingredients.

Prioritize Restaurants with Wild-Caught and Sustainable Seafood

Seafood can be a tricky category when dining out. Look for restaurants that serve wild-caught fish or sustainably farmed seafood. Phrases like "wild-caught Alaskan salmon" or "line-caught swordfish" indicate that the restaurant values both the environment and your health by avoiding overfished species and unsustainable practices.

How to Spot Seafood Sources on the Menu

- Look for labels like "wild caught," "line caught," or "sustainably farmed."
- Menus that mention organizations like the Marine Stewardship Council (MSC) or Monterey Bay Aquarium Seafood Watch are also a good sign that the restaurant is committed to sustainable seafood practices.

Wild-caught fish are often lower in contaminants like mercury and have a better nutritional profile, with higher levels of omega-3 fatty acids. Sustainable practices also help protect ocean ecosystems.

Seek Out Farm-to-Table and Locally Sourced Restaurants

Farm-to-table dining means that the restaurant sources most, if not all, of its ingredients locally and seasonally. These restaurants often have close relationships with farmers and purveyors, ensuring that the produce, meat, and dairy they serve are fresh and responsibly sourced.

How to Spot Local Relationships on the Menu

- Menus may feature seasonal dishes and change frequently based on what's available.
- Look for terms like "locally sourced," "farm-to-table," "seasonal," and "from our local farmers."
- Some restaurants even have partnerships with local farms and will list them on the menu or their website.

Farm-to-table dining supports local agriculture, reduces the environmental footprint of food transportation, and ensures you're getting the freshest, most nutrient-dense ingredients possible.

Avoid Restaurants That Rely on Mass-Produced Ingredients

Places that don't mention where their ingredients come from or use vague terms like "fresh" or "all-natural" without specifics may not be prioritizing quality. Chain restaurants often rely on mass-produced, prepackaged ingredients that lack the nutritional value and care you'd find at a restaurant committed to quality sourcing.

How to Spot Mass-Produced Ingredients on the Menu

- Lack of detail about ingredient sourcing
- Overly large menus with an extensive list of dishes, indicating the use of preprepared or frozen items
- Generic descriptions without mention of specific farms, regions, or sustainable practices

Restaurants that aren't transparent about their ingredients often prioritize cost over quality, which can mean lower nutritional value and a higher likelihood of additives and preservatives.

Dining Out with Confidence

Choosing the right restaurant can make all the difference in your dining experience. By selecting places that proudly list the source of their ingredients, serve wild-caught and sustainably farmed seafood, and embrace farm-to-table practices, you can enjoy delicious meals that align with your health and ethical values.

Next time you're planning to dine out, take a few minutes to research the restaurant's menu online. Look for options that offer grilled, steamed, broiled, or baked dishes instead of fried ones. Call ahead to ask about their sourcing practices. You'll not only enjoy a better meal but also support businesses that are committed to high-quality, sustainable dining.

Additional Tips for Dining Out

- **Watch portion sizes.** Restaurant portions can be much larger than what you need. Share dishes, order appetizers as your main course, or take half of your meal to go.
- **Focus on fiber and protein.** Ensure each meal includes fiber and protein to help you feel full longer on fewer calories. This combination is crucial for maintaining a healthy weight and satiety.
- **Avoid creamy sauces.** Ask for dressings on the side to control how much you consume.
- **Stay hydrated.** Drink plenty of water throughout the day. It helps with digestion and can prevent you from mistaking thirst for hunger.
- **Avoid empty calories.** Skip sugary cocktails, cold bread baskets (it's harder to say no to a warm freshly baked bread!), and high-calorie appetizers. Opt for water, ask for lemon, unsweetened tea, hot water with fresh mint leaves (fresh mint tea), or a small salad to start.

Healthy Foodie Dining While Traveling

Traveling adds another layer of challenge to choosing the healthiest and most nutritious options for your meals. Try these tips for sticking to your best options 80 percent of the time.

- **Pack healthy snacks.** Bring nutritious snacks like unsalted nuts, salmon, or beef jerky without added sugar, roasted chickpeas, or no-sugar-added protein bars. My favorites are Fasting Bar by Prolon and David Protein Bar, formulated by leading longevity experts. This prevents you from grabbing unhealthy options on the go.

- **Stay hydrated.** Stay hydrated by carrying a water bottle with you, especially when flying or sightseeing. Having a water bottle serves as a reminder to stay hydrated and prevents prolonged periods without drinking. Avoid sugary drinks and be cautious with juices and flavored waters as they may contain hidden sugars and artificial ingredients.
- **Don't skip meals.** Stick to regular mealtimes to keep your energy levels stable and avoid overeating later in the day. Aim for two to three meals a day to keep blood sugar stable.
- **Choose wisely at buffets.** Go for proteins and fiber first, fill up half of your plate with colorful vegetables, and then add healthy carbs from Chapter 5. Avoid creamy dishes, deep-fried tempura foods, and high-calorie desserts.
- **Visit local grocery stores.** Stock your hotel room with healthy options like nuts, plain yogurt, fresh fruit, hummus, or precut vegetables.
- **Stay active.** Remember that regular movement is far more beneficial than sitting for two days and then sweating at the gym for one hour. Stay active with dance breaks, stretching, walking, using stairs instead of elevators, and doing simple exercises in your hotel room.

My favorite is the Five Tibetan Yoga Rites, which require no equipment—so there's absolutely no excuse not to do them! The Five Tibetan Yoga Rites are a series of simple exercises designed to improve strength, flexibility, and energy flow. Each rite involves specific movements, such as spinning to activate energy centers, leg raises to strengthen the core, and backbends to enhance spinal flexibility. These exercises take just ten to fifteen minutes a day and are believed to balance the body's energy systems, making them an excellent practice for overall vitality and well-being.

When in Rome

An interesting note for international travelers: As many gluten-sensitive people have found, wheat products are different in Europe and may not aggravate their health to the same extent as they do in the United States. I can't tell you how many clients have shared that they could never eat pastries at home without feeling awful, but a croissant in France is no problem! That's because European wheat is less processed and genetically modified than American wheat, which has much higher levels of gluten. If you're traveling to Europe, feel free to enjoy a trip to the boulangerie or pizzeria—just go slow, notice how your body is tolerating it, and remember to eat protein and high-fiber vegetables first.

Now that we've covered what to eat and how to eat it—no matter where you are or what life throws your way—in the next chapter, I introduce the concept of nutrition cycling. You'll learn how your food intake should align with what your body is experiencing at any given time, embodying the true essence of the Foodie Diet, which is rooted in bio-individuality!

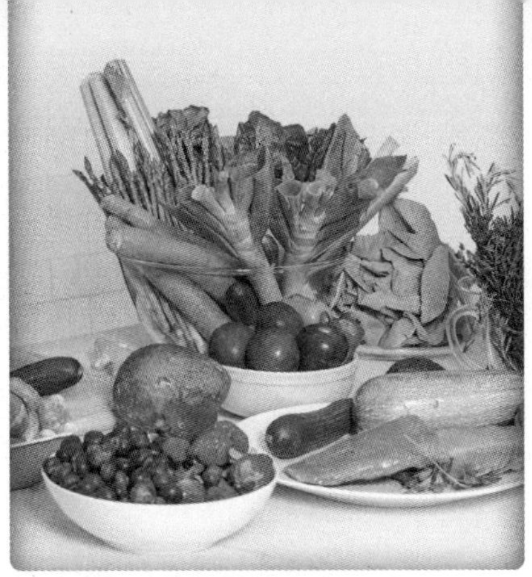

Chapter 7

Feed Your Hormone Balance: A Woman's Guide to Hormonal Nutrition

Let me start this chapter by sharing my personal journey. I intimately understand the struggle with PMS cravings and painful periods. While studying nutrition at NYU and working with countless female clients, I discovered something transformative: Our nutrition needs follow a natural twenty-eight-day rhythm that most diet plans completely ignore.

If you're a woman who wants to lose weight and feel confident in your body—whether that means liking what you see in the mirror or feeling great in your favorite clothes—it might be time to stop chasing one-size-fits-all diets and start tuning into the wisdom of your own body. It's time to honor your feminine biology and work with it, not against it.

Why One-Size-Fits-All Diets Fail Women

Women's bodies operate on a sophisticated hormonal schedule that affects everything from energy levels to nutrient requirements. What works during your follicular phase might be counterproductive during your luteal phase, yet most nutrition advice treats every day as identical.

Throughout the menstrual cycle, women experience natural fluctuations in their metabolism, affecting how their bodies process carbohydrates and utilize protein. These variations influence energy levels and nutrient needs at different phases of the cycle.

Research indicates that carbohydrate utilization varies across the menstrual cycle. A study published in the *British Journal of Nutrition* found that carbohydrate utilization was lower during the early follicular phase, suggesting hormonal influences on energy substrate metabolism.

Additionally, hormonal changes can impact protein metabolism. Elevated progesterone levels during the luteal phase may increase protein catabolism, affecting protein requirements. Understanding these metabolic variations is crucial for tailoring nutritional strategies to support women's health throughout their menstrual cycles.

Also, some researchers have found that intermittent fasting can help with PMS symptoms and may actually improve female health and fertility. This may be due to the improvement of insulin sensitivity and a reduction in glucose and insulin levels.

The menstrual cycle has four phases: menstruation, follicular phase, ovulation, and the luteal phase. Hormones fluctuate during these phases and affect your mood, energy, and appetite. The four weeks of the female cycle differ dramatically, so eating the right foods (and knowing when to eat them) and listening to your body can optimize your health and fitness throughout the month.

Nature created us perfectly in sync with the rhythms of light and darkness, waking and sleeping, hunger and satiety—and this same intelligence applies to the body's monthly cycle. That's why, throughout the one-month cycle, there are ideal times to focus on detoxification with more plants, and other times when consuming animal protein can help balance hormones and prevent cravings for junk food or sugar.

If you are feeling confused about where to begin, don't worry. I created a solution for you! To have a better understanding and more control over your body, be a woman with a cycle plan.

The Four Phases: Your Body's Natural Rhythm

1. Menstruation (Days 1–5):
   - Nutrient needs focus on iron replenishment and anti-inflammatory support
   - Energy requirements often lower
   - Body primed for gentle detoxification
2. Follicular Phase (Days 6–14):
   - Rising estrogen supports lean protein utilization
   - Optimal time for plant-based eating
   - Enhanced insulin sensitivity
3. Ovulation (Days 14–17):
   - Peak energy levels
   - Highest nutrient absorption
   - Ideal time for nutrient-dense foods

4. Luteal Phase (Days 18–28):
    - Increased caloric needs (up to 300 extra calories)
    - Higher protein requirements
    - Strategic carbohydrate timing crucial for preventing cravings

Cycle-Syncing: Your Monthly Cycle Plan

WEEK 1: MENSTRUATION

Around days 1 through 6 of your menstrual cycle when you're bleeding

INNER WINTER

This is the first day you begin bleeding, and it's week one of your cycle. It usually begins on day 1 of the moon cycle as well. The bleeding phase of your cycle is when your energy and hormones are at an all-time low.

The scientific rationale behind treating menstruation as your "inner winter" lies in the dramatic drop in both estrogen and progesterone. During certain phases of the menstrual cycle, inflammatory markers may rise while metabolic rate typically fluctuates, often increasing during the luteal phase due to hormonal changes like elevated progesterone.

EXERCISE. Hibernation and rest are words that accurately characterize what this phase is about for a woman, but a spiritual element is also woven in. This is the week to be gentle with your body.

Research demonstrates that high-intensity exercise during menstruation can increase inflammatory markers. Practice yin (restorative) yoga or meditation, or get out in nature and walk while reflecting and taking deep breaths, which helps reduce prostaglandin production, the compounds responsible for menstrual cramps.

SELF-CARE. Winter is not a time to give to others but to ourselves. Learning to be self-loving during this time is the healthiest behavior we can adopt for ourselves and our families. I recommend taking baths, having movie nights at home, spending the days alone creating or writing/reading, sleeping, and being in nature.

NUTRITION AND FOOD. Eat foods with magnesium to help with irritability, cramps, constipation, and trouble sleeping. These include quinoa, oats, pumpkin seeds, cashews, and almonds. Foods rich in iron will help replenish blood and iron lost through menses; add beef liver, oysters, or kale. Don't forget to eat vitamin C–containing foods for better iron absorption, such as broccoli (make a bone broth–based broccoli soup), strawberries, red peppers, and mango. Drink chamomile or raspberry leaf tea to balance hormones and alleviate cramps.

Your body's need for iron increases by a factor of two to three during menstruation. Here is what I recommend:

- **MORNING.** Start with a magnesium-rich breakfast (½ cup quinoa + 2 tablespoons pumpkin seeds = 150 mg magnesium) or make an Extralicious Antioxidant Berry Smoothie Parfait with beets from Chapter 9.
- **LUNCH.** An iron-boosting combination (3 ounces beef liver and a kale salad with vitamin C–rich red peppers = 12 mg iron), and make sure to pair it with Waist-Slimming Red Cabbage Salad from Chapter 9.
- **DINNER.** Anti-inflammatory focus on bone broth–based soups, like the Simple Bone Broth–Based Broccoli Soup recipe in Chapter 9.

Client Case Study: Sarah—Relief from Cramps and Fatigue

Sarah, a thirty-two-year-old executive, struggled with debilitating cramps and fatigue during menstruation. By implementing this protocol—particularly the combination of 400 mg magnesium glycinate supplementation and iron-rich foods with vitamin C—her pain levels decreased from 9 out of 10 to 3 out of 10 within two cycles.

Fasting and timing. For days 1 to 6, you can practice circadian fasting for at least twelve to fourteen hours, and by the end of the week, restart higher-intensity workouts if desired. The twelve- to fourteen-hour circadian fasting window aligns with natural insulin sensitivity patterns during menstruation. Clinical studies show this timing can reduce PMS symptoms by 47 percent through improved glucose regulation.

Circadian Fasting

According to doctors at UCLA Health, "In the circadian diet, you eat during a 12-hour window—typically between 7:00AM and 7:00PM—and fast during the other 12 hours. Meal sizes are flipped, with breakfast the largest meal of the day and dinner the smallest. That 12-hour nightly fast eliminates after-dinner snacking and midnight raids on the fridge."

Supplement protocol. According to Hormone University, magnesium levels drop by up to 50 percent during menstruation. Deficiency in magnesium can exacerbate menstrual cramps and other symptoms. Supplementation has been shown to reduce the severity and duration of menstrual cramps.

5-Hydroxytryptophan (5-HTP) and Vitamin B_6 for PMS, Mood, and Energy Support

Studies suggest that 5-HTP, a precursor to serotonin, may alleviate PMS-related mood disturbances. Other research suggests that supplementation with vitamin B_6 may do the same. Vitamin B_6 acts as a cofactor in serotonin synthesis, as serotonin is a precursor to melatonin, the hormone responsible for sleep regulation. However, 5-HTP should be used with professional guidance as it can interact with other medications and affect serotonin levels. While it's available over the counter, it's best limited to the luteal and menstrual phases of the cycle to target PMS-specific symptoms effectively.

SUPPLEMENT PROTOCOL RECOMMENDATIONS FOR MENSTRUATION

Some of my clients report a reduction in cramping when following this protocol.

- Start the morning with a high-quality **B-complex supplement.** I've found timing matters significantly here—taking B vitamins first thing supports energy production when your body needs it most. For my clients experiencing significant menstrual fatigue, I recommend focusing on B_6 (50 to 100 mg) and B_{12}, which work synergistically to support energy and mood.
- **Magnesium** becomes particularly crucial during this phase. I recommend splitting the dose: Take your first serving

with lunch and another before bed. This approach provides steady support for muscle relaxation while helping to reduce cramping. Many of my clients report better sleep with this evening dose.

- For mood support during this vulnerable time, 5-HTP can be particularly beneficial when taken in the evening (50 to 100 mg). However, I always caution my clients to start with the lower dose to assess their response.

Pro Tip from a Dietitian

Never take these supplements on an empty stomach. I recommend pairing your morning B-complex with a protein-rich breakfast, and taking magnesium with meals containing healthy fats for optimal absorption. If using CBD oil for additional comfort, time it with your evening magnesium dose.

WEEK 2: FOLLICULAR PHASE

Around days 7 to 13 when you're in the preovulation phase

INNER SPRING

Ahhh, spring! It's the second week of your cycle, when you reemerge after a period of hibernation from the world. Think rebirth, renewal, a fresh start—cleansed, energized, and happy. As a woman moves into her inner-spring phase, she's ready to get back into the world and take on new projects. This is when you can start planning and organizing your month. During this phase, rising estrogen optimizes glucose metabolism and increases insulin sensitivity by up to

30 percent. Muscle protein synthesis peaks, making it ideal for strength training and muscle recovery.

EXERCISE. This week is the best week for high-intensity workouts and maximum training efforts, so try a spin class or strength workout. Peak muscle glycogen storage capacity occurs during this phase, so train like an athlete. During this phase, your body becomes remarkably efficient at building and repairing muscle tissue. Studies demonstrate that anaerobic capacity and muscle strength are greatest during the follicular phase of the menstrual cycle, when estrogen levels peak. This is nature's gift—a time when estrogen's anticatabolic effects enhance recovery and reduce muscle damage.

During the follicular phase, your body naturally recovers faster and performs more efficiently—making it an ideal time to push your limits with higher-intensity workouts like spin, interval training, or strength circuits. Research shows women experience better neuromuscular coordination and reduced inflammation during this phase, helping them train harder with less strain.

SELF-CARE. During your spring phase, estrogen rises and energy levels come back. This is an optimal time for dedication to projects, reading and researching, learning, and performing physical tasks. It's the best time to take on a challenge.

NUTRITION AND FOOD. Nutritionally, this phase presents a unique opportunity. This is the perfect time to eat carbohydrate-rich foods because insulin sensitivity is at its peak. Quinoa salad (see the recipe in Chapter 9) and sweet potatoes are a great complex carbohydrate combination packed with vitamins A, C, and B_6, calcium, magnesium, potassium, and iron. Eat foods that metabolize estrogen for hormone balance, including sprouted and fermented foods like broccoli sprouts, kimchi, and sauerkraut. Now is also a fine time to try a cleanse and incorporate vegan or vegetarian days for a detox because you naturally have enough energy.

FASTING AND TIMING. The follicular phase offers the perfect window for extending your fasting period to fourteen to sixteen hours. This is the time to try a push fast—something one to two hours longer than usual, which can be up to sixteen hours. This is a time when you feel most disciplined and have no food cravings, which is why any restrictions feel easier to accomplish. You can also increase your carbohydrates so you have the energy to work out. Your insulin sensitivity is excellent during this time. Research shows this timing can increase growth hormone production by up to 1,200 percent and enhance cellular autophagy markers. Most importantly, women report feeling naturally less hungry during this phase, making it easier to maintain a longer fasting window.

Client Case Study: Strength and Body Composition

Emma, a twenty-eight-year-old athlete, transformed her training approach by aligning her workouts with her follicular phase. Within just three months, she increased her strength by 15 percent, experienced significantly faster recovery times, and saw noticeable improvements in body composition. Her success highlights the power of working with—rather than against—your body's natural hormonal rhythms.

SUPPLEMENTS FOR THE FOLLICULAR PHASE

During the follicular phase, your body's enhanced nutrient absorption capabilities create a perfect window for targeted supplementation. Specific nutrients can amplify the natural metabolic advantages of this phase. Your primary focus should be on supplements that support estrogen metabolism and energy production.

- B-complex vitamins become particularly crucial, with studies showing that B_6 and B_{12} support the increased energy demands of this phase. I recommend 50 mg of B_6 and 1,000 mcg of methylated B_{12} taken in the morning to match your body's natural cortisol rhythm.
- Antioxidant support becomes essential during this high-energy phase. Glutathione precursors and NAC (N-Acetyl Cysteine) at 600 mg daily support your body's natural detoxification processes, which are naturally enhanced during this time. Research published in the *Journal of Clinical Medicine* demonstrates that NAC supplementation during the follicular phase can improve cellular energy production.
- If you are into higher-intensity workouts, adding BCAAs in a 2:1:1 ratio has shown to improve exercise recovery and reduce muscle soreness. The optimal timing is thirty minutes pre-workout or immediately post-workout.
- Magnesium requirements decrease slightly from your menstrual phase, but maintaining a baseline of 200 to 300 mg daily, preferably in glycinate form, supports this time's increased energy production and muscle recovery demands.Green tea extract (standardized for EGCG) taken in the morning (matcha is my favorite) can enhance the natural

fat-burning potential of this phase while supporting healthy estrogen metabolism. Clinical studies suggest 300 to 400 mg EGCG during this phase optimizes metabolic flexibility.

WEEK 3: OVULATION/LUTEAL PHASE

Around days 14 to 21, during your ovulation phase

INNER SUMMER

This phase, often referred to as "inner summer," is when things begin heating up—literally and metaphorically. During this third week of the menstrual cycle, ovulation occurs, typically around day 14. Body temperature rises due to progesterone, testosterone levels will be at their highest, and sex drive is at its highest. This is also a time of heightened energy, creativity, and social connectivity!

EXERCISE RECOMMENDATIONS. During the ovulation phase, energy levels are more outward and expressive, making it an ideal time for activities like strength training, Pilates, and barre. However, with elevated body temperature due to ovulation, be cautious of overheating and avoid overly intense workouts. Instead, focus on controlled movements that build strength while maintaining balance. Research indicates that a higher body temperature can also affect hydration and endurance, so ensure adequate hydration during exercise.

SELF-CARE. Ovulation is a time for connection and community. You may feel more social and motivated to nurture relationships, host gatherings, or provide support to loved ones. This is also an excellent phase for deepening intimacy with your partner—just remember that fertility is heightened, so take precautions if pregnancy isn't the goal. Interestingly, I've heard some female health experts suggest that ovulation is when women feel their most powerful—more confident and energized—and is the best time to ask for what you want, such as discussing a raise at work or having meaningful conversations with your partner. Try it!

NUTRITION AND FOOD. During this phase, focus on higher-protein, lower-carbohydrate foods to support hormonal balance and maintain stable blood sugar levels. Insulin sensitivity begins to decrease as the luteal phase progresses, making it crucial to prioritize nutrient-dense, anti-inflammatory foods. Recommended proteins include grass-fed steak, chicken, turkey, beef liver, oily fish (salmon, mackerel, sardines), and shrimp. Complement these with anti-inflammatory and detoxifying foods:

- **Nuts and seeds**—almonds and walnuts
- **Spices**—ginger and turmeric
- **Vegetables**—broccoli, kale, and mushrooms
- **Fruits**—blueberries, pomegranates, cranberries, cherries, and grapefruit

These foods help detoxify excess estrogen and provide the necessary micronutrients to support ovulation and hormone production. For example, cruciferous vegetables like kale contain indole-3-carbinol, which supports estrogen metabolism.

SUPPLEMENTS FOR THE OVULATION PHASE

Around days 14 to 21, your body experiences its peak hormonal activity. As a gut health dietitian, I've developed specific supplement protocols to support healthy ovulation.

- **Omega-3 fatty acids,** particularly EPA and DHA, become especially important during this time. For my clients, I recommend either high-quality fish oil or algae-based supplements for those following a plant-based diet. Timing matters here—take these with your largest meal of the day to maximize absorption.

- **Magnesium** becomes your best friend during ovulation. I prefer magnesium glycinate for my clients due to its superior absorption and gentle effect on the digestive system. Many of them report better energy levels and reduced cramping when taking it in the evening.
- A quality **probiotic** can make a significant difference—I've seen remarkable improvements in my clients' hormone-related symptoms when we focus on gut health. Look for multistrain formulas that include both *Lactobacillus and Bifidobacterium* species.
- **Ashwagandha** is known for its adaptogenic properties, helping manage stress, especially for women engaging in regular exercise. Chronic stress can disrupt ovulatory hormones, so ashwagandha is a valuable addition during this phase.

Pro Tip from a Dietitian

Pair your supplements strategically with meals. Fat-soluble nutrients like vitamin D need healthy fats for optimal absorption. I recommend taking them with foods like avocado, eggs, or olive oil–dressed salads.

Through years of clinical practice, I've found that this targeted approach helps support your body's natural rhythms during ovulation. However, remember that supplement needs are highly individual—what works beautifully for one person might need adjustment for another.

FASTING AND TIMING. The luteal phase is an ideal time to establish consistency with a 16:8 intermittent fasting protocol (fasting for sixteen hours with an eight-hour eating window). This approach can help stabilize blood sugar levels and optimize energy use. However, fasting should always be personalized, especially for women with high activity levels or adrenal fatigue, to avoid exacerbating stress on the body.

By understanding and aligning with the hormonal shifts of your ovulation phase, you can maximize your physical and emotional well-being while supporting long-term healthy metabolism and hormonal balance.

WEEK 4: LUTEAL PHASE

Around days 22 to 29

INNER FALL (WINDING DOWN AGAIN)

The fourth week of your cycle is when the body and mind naturally begin to wind down. If you start becoming more mindful and paying more attention, you'll notice how you may feel more inward focused this week, craving solitude and becoming easily agitated by excessive demands. Personally, I schedule my life around this phase, intentionally setting aside extra time for self-care and reflection as my period approaches. Honoring this inward shift is an act of self-love and resilience, and I encourage you to do the same.

The late luteal phase is often associated with PMS. The week before your period, your body is most vulnerable to stress. Estrogen levels drop significantly, heightening cortisol sensitivity (our stress hormone) and amplifying emotional and physical vulnerabilities. This heightened sensitivity makes it essential to prioritize gentleness, self-compassion, and balance in your daily routine.

EXERCISE. During this week, try gentle exercise and restorative activities, like swimming, Pilates, or dance class—nothing too hard or stressful. Take time off and avoid strenuous workouts as your body is more prone to stress during this time. Breathwork, meditation, and spending time outdoors or in nature can help regulate cortisol levels and support a sense of calm.

SELF-CARE. Listen to your body during the fall phase. You may feel inspired and want to pursue creative ideas. This is a wonderful time to create strategic ideas for your business or career and assert yourself. However, it's equally important to acknowledge and honor moments when you feel down or fatigued, so treat yourself with extra compassion this week, and give your body a little rest. Schedule a monthly spa day and a massage, and spend some time in nature. Have some really good self-care time to recharge. Nurturing your mind and body can help alleviate stress and enhance your mood.

NUTRITION AND FOOD. To prevent food cravings, make sure to include some healthy fats and 2 to 3 ounces of high-quality protein—such as steak, beef or chicken livers, or vegetarian alternatives like tempeh, tofu, lentils, or hemp seeds at every meal. This is not a time to diet or limit your food intake. Make sure to eat enough fiber-rich foods like green leafy vegetables with protein; fats like avocado, olives, and ghee; and full-fat dairy products like yogurt and kefir. Snack on olives, salmon or beef jerky, dark chocolate, walnuts, cherries, and pomegranates. Magnesium-rich foods help fight fatigue and prevent low libido: quinoa, oats, lentils, black beans, spinach, kale, cashews, pumpkin seeds, almonds, and dark chocolate (70-plus percent cacao). Add magnesium-rich pumpkin seeds and hemp seeds to your salad or smoothie.

Aim to have high-protein meals and incorporate ingredients like soothing peppermint tea or chai latte with no caffeine, which will satisfy your cravings without adding a high sugar load.

FASTING AND TIMING. This is not the time to push your body with high-intensity workouts or prolonged fasting. Avoid unnecessary stressors and focus on relaxation and recovery. If you can't take a break from fasting entirely, reduce your fasting window to twelve hours instead of your usual sixteen to eighteen. This phase calls for extra self-care and lighter, restorative activities to support your body's natural needs.

SUPPLEMENTS. During the luteal phase, your body's nutrient requirements shift. Magnesium needs often increase to support muscle relaxation and minimize cramping. For sleep support and hormone balance, several natural options can be helpful. Evening primrose oil provides gamma-linolenic acid, which helps modulate prostaglandin production. CBD and GABA-supporting herbs may promote relaxation and better sleep quality when discomfort peaks.

Pro Tip from a Dietitian

Start with magnesium glycinate at dinner, as this form is gentle on the stomach and has good absorption. If using evening primrose oil, take it with a meal containing healthy fats for optimal absorption. Always introduce one supplement at a time to understand how your body responds, and remember that supplements should complement, not replace, a nutrient-rich diet, particularly during this phase.

Seed Cycling: Nature's Hormonal Support

Seed cycling has emerged as a natural approach to support hormonal balance throughout your menstrual cycle. While scientific research on seed cycling is limited, the practice leverages the nutrient-rich profiles of seeds like flax, pumpkin, sesame, and sunflower, which contain compounds thought to influence hormone metabolism.

How It Works

Seed cycling aligns with the two main phases of the menstrual cycle: the follicular phase (days 1 to 14) and the luteal phase (days 15 to 28).

- During the follicular phase, women consume 1 tablespoon each of ground pumpkin and flax seeds daily. Pumpkin seeds are rich in zinc, which supports progesterone production, while flax seeds contain lignans that help bind to and eliminate excess estrogen.
- In the luteal phase, the focus shifts to sesame and sunflower seeds, with women consuming 1 tablespoon of each per day. Sesame seeds provide lignans that support progesterone production, while sunflower seeds offer selenium, an essential nutrient for liver function and hormone metabolism.

Potential Benefits

Though evidence is primarily anecdotal, seed cycling may offer several potential benefits:

- **Hormonal balance.** Nutrients in the seeds may help align with natural hormonal fluctuations, alleviating menstrual irregularities and PMS symptoms.
- **Improved fertility.** By supporting healthy ovulation and

hormone metabolism, seed cycling may enhance reproductive health.

- **PMS relief.** The seeds' nutrient profiles may reduce bloating, mood swings, and cramps.
- **Digestive health.** High fiber content supports digestion and regular bowel movements.
- **Anti-inflammatory effects.** Seeds' anti-inflammatory properties can help mitigate hormonal imbalance–related inflammation.

Pro Tip from a Dietitian

Store seeds in the refrigerator, and grind them fresh daily to preserve their delicate nutrients. I recommend adding them to morning smoothies or sprinkling over salads for easy integration into your daily routine. Try Beeya Wellness formulas with black sesame seeds designed to support a natural cycle with seed formulas for two phases of the cycle.

Hormonal Changes and Menopause Support

Menopause is a challenging time for many women, especially because of symptoms like unwanted or stubborn weight gain, which often leaves my clients feeling frustrated and defeated. They come to my office in despair, saying things like, "I feel like I've lost touch with my body. Nothing works anymore. I don't have any control over it. Whatever I try doesn't work for me—no portion control, no high-protein diet. Please help!"

This phase of life brings significant hormonal shifts that affect metabolism, insulin sensitivity, and muscle mass, often making traditional weight-loss strategies ineffective. However, understanding these changes and tailoring a specific approach to nutrition, gut health, and hormonal support can make a profound difference. As a gut health dietitian, I've seen firsthand how addressing underlying imbalances—such as beta-glucuronidase enzyme levels and hormonal detoxification—can empower women to regain control of their health and achieve long-term results.

I emphasize the importance of understanding the role of the gut microbiome in managing hormonal changes during menopause. One critical factor is the enzyme beta-glucuronidase, produced by gut bacteria, which plays a key role in hormone metabolism and detoxification. During menopause, low levels of beta-glucuronidase, often identified through comprehensive stool testing, can impair the body's ability to eliminate excess hormones, particularly estrogen, potentially leading to imbalances and exacerbated symptoms like weight gain, mood swings, hot flashes, and even insomnia.

To support healthy beta-glucuronidase activity and improve hormone detoxification, focus on foods rich in soluble and insoluble fiber, such as cruciferous vegetables (broccoli, kale, cauliflower), apples, carrots, flaxseeds, and psyllium husk. Cruciferous vegetables, in particular, contain indole-3-carbinol, a compound shown to promote estrogen metabolism. Probiotic-rich foods like yogurt, kimchi, and sauerkraut enhance gut bacterial diversity, supporting enzyme activity and overall hormone balance.

Pro Tip from a Dietitian

For maximum benefit, lightly steam cruciferous vegetables to enhance their digestibility while preserving their nutrient content. Pair them with healthy fats, like olive oil or avocado, as well as mustard seeds, to improve nutrient absorption. Make sure that at least half of your plate is filled with vegetables!

Include polyphenol-rich foods like berries, green tea, and pomegranate, which help reduce inflammation and improve gut health. Healthy fats from omega-3-rich fish, nuts, and seeds stabilize blood sugar levels and combat insulin resistance, which are common challenges during menopause. Foods high in calcium (leafy greens, sardines, almonds) and vitamin D are also key for maintaining bone density and hormonal balance.

Scientific studies indicate that high-fiber diets, rich in phytonutrients and anti-inflammatory compounds, can improve hormone metabolism and reduce menopausal symptoms. Combining these dietary changes with regular physical activity and stress management techniques offers a holistic approach to navigating menopause with improved energy, mood, and overall health.

Testosterone and Longevity: The Role of Nutrition

While I'm not a hormone specialist, my role as a dietitian is to help you understand how nutrition directly impacts your testosterone levels—a crucial hormone for men and women that affects energy, mood, bone density, and overall vitality. Let me share what I've learned through years of clinical practice.

Think of testosterone production like building a house—you need the right materials. In my practice, I focus on three key nutritional pillars: zinc-rich foods, vitamin D, and healthy fats. Oysters top my list for zinc content; just six oysters provide more zinc than you need in a day. For clients who don't enjoy oysters, I recommend pumpkin seeds and grass-fed beef as alternatives.

Zinc is an essential mineral for testosterone production and hormonal health. Zinc supports the enzymatic processes involved in synthesizing testosterone and maintaining optimal levels. For an extra mineral boost, prioritize zinc-rich foods—also including chickpeas and cashews—especially if you haven't included them in earlier meals.

Pro Tip from a Dietitian

Pair zinc-rich foods with vitamin C sources like bell peppers or citrus fruits to enhance absorption and support overall hormonal health.

For women, particularly during and after menopause, maintaining optimal testosterone becomes crucial for preserving muscle mass and bone density. I've seen remarkable improvements in my female clients' energy and vitality when we focus on anti-inflammatory foods and optimal protein intake at every meal, as discussed in Chapter 5.

Timing matters. Protein consumption after strength training, combined with adequate zinc intake, supports your body's natural testosterone production. I recommend spacing zinc-rich foods throughout the day for optimal absorption rather than consuming them all at once.

Pro Tip from a Dietitian

Hormones and the endocrine system are deeply connected to nutrient intake. I recommend that every woman age thirty-five and older start with the foundation—learning about your unique hormonal balance and metabolism from the tools described in Chapter 3. A tailored approach that accounts for your bio-individuality is the most effective path to sustained hormonal health.

Sleep quality is nonnegotiable for hormone production. I guide my clients to create what I call a hormone-supporting evening routine: finishing dinner at least three hours before bedtime and including magnesium-rich foods like pumpkin seeds or leafy greens with dinner to support quality sleep.

Seasonality: Nature's Guide to Optimal Nutrition

In my practice as a functional medicine dietitian, I emphasize aligning nutrition with nature's rhythms. Seasonal eating isn't just a trend. It's deeply rooted in traditional wisdom and modern nutritional science, and it can be adapted to any region, including warm climates like Florida where seasonal shifts are more subtle but still meaningful.

Summer's bounty of water-rich fruits and vegetables provides natural hydration when we need it most. Autumn's focus is on food preservation. Winter's root vegetables and fatty fish offer sustained energy and nutrients when our bodies require more insulation and support our increased need for calories and nutrients. This isn't just about food availability—it's about matching our nutrition to our body's changing seasonal needs. And when spring arrives, lighter eating returns.

Seasonal Eating in My Childhood

Growing up on my grandparents' farm in rural Russia, I experienced this firsthand. My family's meals flowed with the seasons. Summer meant vibrant salads with garden-fresh tomatoes and fragrant herbs picked minutes before dinner. As autumn approached, our kitchen transformed into a preservation workshop where we would ferment and pickle vegetables to prepare for the winter ahead.

Winter called for heartier fare. Root vegetables, fermented cabbage, and rich meats provided the sustenance needed during cold months. These warming foods naturally support our body's increased need for calories and nutrients during colder seasons. What's fascinating is how this aligns perfectly with our metabolism's seasonal shifts. Comfort food cravings are on the rise during this time, and as much as I love vegetables, I do not mean only salads. During the winter, I recommend what I call "temperature-treated vegetables"—lightly sautéed, steamed, cooked, baked, or sous vide and soups. Lots of easy recipes are in Chapter 9.

By spring, our pantry would be nearly empty, leading to a natural period of lighter eating—what many cultures recognize as a fasting or detox period. Today, I see how this traditional wisdom mirrors our body's natural detoxification cycles. This parallels the Christian tradition of Lent and the Muslim tradition of Ramadan, and the benefits extend beyond spiritual practice to physiological renewal.

Pro Tip from a Dietitian

Start small with seasonal eating. Visit your local farmers' market and choose what's abundant. In winter, focus on warming foods like roasted root vegetables and hearty soups. Come summer, embrace cooling foods—think cucumber mint salads and fresh berries. Your body naturally craves what it needs each season. Learning to listen to these cues is key.

How to Eat to Balance Hormones: Your Calendar for Wellness

As we've explored in this chapter, supporting your hormones isn't about quick fixes or miracle supplement. It's about understanding how nutrition, timing, and lifestyle work together to support your body's natural rhythms.

From our deep dive into cycle syncing and menopause support to understanding testosterone's role in longevity, one theme remains constant: *Your food choices directly impact your hormonal health.* Whether you're dealing with monthly cycles, navigating menopause, or focusing on healthy aging, the foundation always comes back to nutrient-dense whole foods, strategic timing, and listening to your body's signals.

Key Takeaways

- Your nutritional needs change throughout your menstrual cycle.
- Timing your meals and supplements matters as much as what you consume.
- Quality protein, healthy fats, and fiber form the foundation of hormone support.
- Sleep and stress management are crucial pieces of the hormone puzzle.
- Seasonal eating supports your body's natural hormonal rhythms.

The next chapter takes these foundational principles and applies them to specific health conditions. I'll share my clinical protocols for healthy weight loss, energy levels, advanced detoxification, healthy hair and vision, women's health concerns, and gut healing—taking everything we've learned about hormones and applying it to targeted therapeutic approaches. Whether you're dealing with autoimmune issues, seeking to optimize your detox pathways, or working to heal your gut, you'll learn how to adapt these hormone-supporting strategies to your unique needs.

Remember, true hormone balance starts with understanding your unique body's needs and honoring them through mindful and educated nutrition choices—through your monthly cycle and the turning of the seasons.

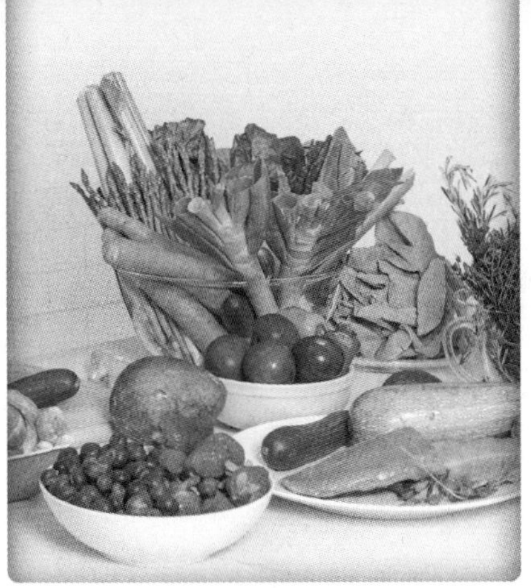

Chapter 8

Feed Your Hunger for Health: Protocols for Specific Health Conditions

In this chapter, I'll dive into specific strategies for weight loss, preventing fatigue, advanced detoxification, cholesterol and hypertension management, gut health, navigating autoimmune conditions, promoting healthy hair and vision, antiaging nutrition, and advanced nutrients for longevity. My fascination with advanced nutrition—the science of how food impacts not just weight but energy, aging, and long-term cellular health—comes from its ability to transform lives, helping my clients alleviate symptoms, reverse underlying conditions, and feel their best.

As a dietitian, my job is to find solutions tailored to each individual, combining the power of targeted protocols, supplements, and dietary strategies. Beyond just managing health issues, my goal is to show you how using food as the foundation of treatment can pave the way for long-term success. By choosing foods and supplements that align with your unique needs, you can build a healthier future and achieve lasting results.

Weight-Loss Medications: A Dietitian's Perspective

Let me address one of the most discussed topics in weight management today: GLP-1 (glucagon-like peptide-1) receptor agonists like Ozempic and Wegovy. Working with clients both before and after using these medications, I've observed their benefits and limitations firsthand.

Research from the *New England Journal of Medicine* demonstrates that GLP-1 agonists can achieve significant weight loss, with participants losing an average of 15 percent body weight over sixty-eight weeks. However, the key question my clients ask remains, "How do I maintain this weight loss naturally?" While these medications can be effective tools, particularly for those with significant weight to lose, the focus still must be on sustainable lifestyle changes. Recent studies show that without behavioral modifications, lost weight can return within two years of discontinuing medication.

As a practitioner, I support medical intervention when appropriate, particularly for clients with a body-mass index over 30 or those with weight-related health complications. For older clients or those with more advanced metabolic decline, medication may be necessary as part of a comprehensive approach. However, for younger or otherwise healthy individuals who can achieve results through lifestyle modification alone, I prioritize building sustainable habits first to prevent nutrient deficiencies and preserve muscle mass. In my work experience, as well as in scientific research, I have seen two critical issues with GLP-1 agonists that require careful attention:

1. First, appetite suppression can lead to some nutrient deficiencies. In my experience, patients on these medications reduce their caloric intake by up to 40 percent, often leading to suboptimal intake of essential nutrients.
2. Second, and perhaps more concerning, is the impact on muscle mass. Research demonstrates that without concurrent resistance training, up to 40 percent of weight loss from GLP-1 agonists can come from lean muscle tissue.

In addition to these concerns, emerging studies have also linked GLP-1 agonists to side effects such as GI distress, potential gallbladder issues, and in rare cases, pancreatitis or thyroid complications.

When my clients choose weight-loss medications, I emphasize that our goal isn't just a lower number on the scale—it's optimal body composition for longevity. This means implementing

- Strategic protein timing for muscle preservation
- Resistance training protocols
- Comprehensive nutrient monitoring
- Mindful food choices, even given a reduced appetite

The science clearly shows that combining medication with proper nutrition and exercise leads to longer-term results in both fat loss and muscle preservation. This comprehensive approach supports not just weight loss but also metabolic health for higher chances of a longer life.

Blood Sugar Management with CGM

Using continuous glucose monitoring (CGM) in my dietetic practice has revolutionized how I approach personalized nutrition. I learned about this technology while in Israel researching the Mediterranean diet. Originally developed for diabetes management, CGM has provided fascinating insights into individual glucose responses and personalized nutrition.

In my practice, I've witnessed significant differences in glycemic responses between couples eating identical meals. I had a husband and wife both wear CGMs while eating the same dinner and dessert. The husband's blood sugar barely moved after eating a slice of chocolate cake, staying within fifteen points of his baseline, while his wife's glucose spiked by over fifty points (mg/dL). This perfectly illustrates research from the Weizmann Institute, showing that two people can have dramatically different glycemic responses to the exact same food, influenced by factors like genetics, gut microbiome composition, and metabolic health.

During the fourteen- to twenty-eight-day CGM period, my clients gain invaluable insights into what's happening beneath the surface—how their food choices directly impact their energy levels and hormonal responses. The immediate feedback, particularly thirty minutes postmeal, is unparalleled. Traditional weight-loss feedback loops, like waiting to see changes on the scale, are often too delayed to create meaningful connections between food choices, cheat meals, and cravings. In contrast, CGM provides real-time data, fostering a clear understanding of how food acts as fuel and supports a healthy metabolism. I call it *the ultimate mind-body bridge!*

Understanding Your Bio-Individuality

When I introduce CGM to my clients, the initial learning curve can be steep due to the constant stream of data received 24/7 for two to four weeks. However, this is where the life-changing insights truly begin. Clients start to see how food affects their energy levels, hormones, and carbohydrate metabolism. It's often eye-opening when they realize that some foods they considered healthy can spike their blood sugar more than foods they thought were unhealthy. For example, one of my Eastern European clients experienced a significant blood sugar spike from tropical foods like mangoes and even watermelon—much higher than from a croissant! This aligns with research on ancestral diet adaptation and reveals how her DNA and ancestral dietary patterns, which lacked tropical fruits and fructose, impacted her glucose response and insulin sensitivity to fructose.

This is where meal composition becomes the focus. No, I didn't tell her to avoid tropical fruits forever. Instead, I taught her how to pair high-carbohydrate foods with healthy fats and proteins for better blood sugar control. For instance, I suggested eating watermelon Mediterranean-style, paired with feta cheese and mint leaves, or enjoying mango on top of a green salad with a protein source. These strategies allow her to enjoy her favorite foods while understanding her unique bio-individuality and maintaining balanced blood sugar levels and improved metabolism. Instead of eliminating foods, I teach strategic food combining. Research shows that adding protein and fat to carbohydrates can reduce glycemic response. This is why I recommend Mediterranean-style cuisine and balanced food-group combinations to support better blood sugar stability while honoring food joy and cultural preferences.

Eating for Weight Loss

It might sound antithetical, but, yes, you have to eat to lose weight! The key is striking the right balance of the three essential levers of nutrition: what you eat, how much you eat, and when you eat. Each plays a critical role in determining long-term success, and pulling them in harmony is where the magic happens.

1. **What you eat.** Focus on nutrient-dense foods from the three major food groups discussed in Chapter 5: proteins, fats, and carbohydrates.

    25 to 35 percent proteins: Include daily a variety of grass-fed meats (beef, bison), pasture-raised poultry (chicken, turkey), and wild-caught fish (salmon, sardines, trout). Add diversity with eggs, seafood (clams, oysters, shrimp), or venison.

    20 to 30 percent healthy fats: Pair proteins with fats like olive oil, ghee, avocados, nuts, and nut butters to support cellular repair and reduce inflammation.

    40 to 50 percent carbohydrates: Prioritize fiber-rich, slow-digesting options like sweet potatoes, quinoa, and cruciferous vegetables to stabilize blood sugar and improve satiety.

Pro Tip from a Dietitian

For breakfast, combine eggs with avocado, or sprinkle nuts over your meal. At dinner, try wild-caught salmon with olive oil and roasted asparagus. Use recipes from Chapter 9.

2. **How much you eat.** Energy balance and caloric intake are key because you can gain weight from eating too much protein, healthy carbs, and fats! To achieve weight loss, focus on creating a slight caloric deficit while maintaining sufficient nutrients to support health.
    - Use a smaller portion and mindful eating practices to avoid overeating.
    - Implement tools like food journaling or tracking apps to monitor possible excessive intake from snacking without becoming overly restrictive. This way, you'll learn how the calories add up. Most people then understand a great deal about caloric density and are able to find more balance later without tracking calories.
    - Adjust portion sizes based on your activity levels, ensuring enough energy for workouts but avoiding excessive caloric intake.
3. **When you eat.** Meal timing can enhance metabolic flexibility and fat loss.
    - For most individuals, strategies like time-restricted eating or intermittent fasting can improve insulin sensitivity and support a caloric deficit.
    - Start with a twelve-hour fasting window (for example, 7:00 PM to 7:00 AM), and gradually expand to fourteen to sixteen hours, if it feels sustainable, by avoiding late dinners.
    - Avoid eating late at night as it can interfere with metabolic efficiency and disrupt circadian rhythms.

By pulling these three levers intentionally—focusing on nutrient quality, portion control, and meal timing—you can create a framework for effective and sustainable weight loss. The foods in Chapter

5 provide a deeper dive into tailoring these principles to your unique needs.

Research-Backed Supplements for Weight Management

There are some specific supplements for weight loss that I often recommend in addition to food and lifestyle recommendations.

Preliminary research suggests that certain probiotic strains may help naturally curb cravings by influencing levels of GLP-1, a hormone involved in appetite regulation. Recent research has identified specific strains that influence GLP-1 production and appetite regulation. The combination of *Akkermansia muciniphila* and specific *Bifidobacterium* strains has shown particular promise in reducing food cravings through multiple mechanisms, including improved gut barrier function and appetite hormone regulation.

Another effective combination for weight loss includes green tea extract (*Camellia sinensis*) paired with cayenne pepper fruit extract, veld grape stem and leaf extract, and other compounds. The combination of EGCG from green tea with capsaicin from cayenne pepper has been shown to increase metabolic rate. For example, the Metabolism+ supplement formula by Mindbodygreen has been researched and formulated to

- **Promote fat metabolism** through catechins in green tea, which enhance thermogenesis and calorie burning.
- **Help burn visceral fat,** which is closely linked to metabolic health risks.
- **Control appetite** by supporting hormonal signals that regulate hunger and satiety.

Incorporating these supplements as part of a holistic weight-loss strategy, alongside balanced nutrition and regular physical activity, can provide an additional edge in achieving and maintaining a healthy body composition.

Feed Your Fatigue

Nutrition plays a fundamental role in determining energy levels within the human body. Once these nutrients enter the cells, the body's metabolism kicks in. Metabolism encompasses all the chemical reactions that occur within the body to maintain life. One of the primary functions of metabolism is to convert macronutrients—carbohydrates, proteins, and fats—into cellular energy (in the form of adenosine triphosphate, or ATP). Fatigue can be a sign of internal imbalances such as low-grade chronic inflammation resulting from food sensitivities. For example, fatigue and brain fog are symptoms of gluten intolerance, which is probably the best-known trigger of food sensitivities.

Inflammation from food sensitivities can disrupt energy production through several mechanisms. Individuals with gluten sensitivity may experience reduced antioxidant levels, including CoQ_{10}, which is essential for mitochondrial function and cellular energy production. Maintaining sufficient CoQ_{10} levels is necessary to support optimal energy metabolism in these individuals.

The best tool we have to identify food sensitivities is a process of careful observation and experimentation. The protocol of removing certain foods believed to cause reactions from the diet for two to four weeks, reintroducing them one by one, and watching for symptoms is the current gold standard to pin down what may be causing symptoms. Such an elimination diet is not high-tech and is far from perfect but it is useful.

Some of the common foods that cause inflammation are anything processed, refined carbohydrates, sugar and high-fructose corn syrup, fried foods, dairy products, artificial additives, and alcohol.

The Science Behind Energy Production

Fatigue isn't just about being tired. It's often a complex interplay of nutrient deficiencies, cellular metabolism, and inflammation. Let me break down the science of how specific nutrient deficiencies directly impact your energy production.

Iron deficiency, particularly when ferritin levels drop below 30 ng/mL, dramatically impairs oxygen transport and ATP production in your mitochondria. Low iron status affects cellular energy production even before clinical anemia develops. When iron levels drop, our cells struggle to produce energy efficiently through the electron transport chain, where iron-dependent enzymes like cytochrome C oxidase play crucial roles in ATP production. This is why fatigue is often one of the first symptoms people notice when their iron levels are suboptimal. Think of B vitamins as your cellular energy team—each playing a unique and crucial role in how your body produces and maintains vitality. Thiamine (B_1) acts as your cellular spark plug, riboflavin (B_2) serves as your energy factory's efficiency expert, and B_{12} becomes increasingly crucial as we age, impacting everything from brain function to DNA repair. This is why I guide my clients to focus on B vitamin–rich foods, particularly after age forty when absorption naturally declines.

The Often-Overlooked Factor

The production of thyroid hormones depends on many key nutrients—including iodine, iron, tyrosine, zinc, selenium, magnesium, and vitamins E, B_2, B_3, B_6, C, and D—which become especially important during menopause and postmenopause, when hormonal shifts can impact thyroid function and metabolism. Thyroid hormones are essential for regulating metabolism. Poor nutrition can impair thyroid function, leading to conditions like hypothyroidism (underactive thyroid) or hyperthyroidism (overactive thyroid), which can both present with fatigue as a symptom.

> Very often, a lack of energy can be resolved by detoxing from inflammatory foods and incorporating more anti-inflammatory options, as described in Chapter 5. I've had people comment and leave reviews for me—even without becoming my clients—sharing stories like this: "I'm a restaurant owner, and I love eating good food. I've never been able to stick to any diet recommendations, but after watching your TEDx Talk on 'The Foods That Love You Back,' I got creative with all the foods you recommended. Now I feel like a brand-new, younger version of myself—I've lost weight and gotten rid of the nagging back pain I've had for years due to inflammatory conditions!" Incorporating more foods from Chapter 5 and building your meals around them can truly help kick-start your metabolism, boost energy, and improve overall health.

Detox to Combat Fatigue

Reduce sugar and alcohol for twenty-one days. Diets high in added sugar can disrupt sleep; elevate blood sugar, inflammation, and insulin levels; and result in dysbiosis and chronic fatigue. Limit all sugar-containing products to an occasional treat to stabilize energy levels and support detoxification naturally.

Eat an anti-inflammatory diet from Chapter 5. Prioritize green and colorful vegetables, antioxidant-rich berries, and omega-3 fatty acids from sources like wild-caught salmon, sardines, and flaxseeds. These foods lower inflammation and improve gut health, essential for sustained energy.

Optimize intake of key nutrients. These include

- **Iron.** Include dark leafy greens like spinach and high-quality protein sources such as grass-fed beef and lentils to support oxygen transport and energy production.
- **B vitamins.** Found in eggs, whole grains, and all animal proteins (meats), these are critical for converting food into energy.
- **Vitamin C.** Add citrus fruits, kiwi, broccoli, and bell peppers to enhance iron absorption, reduce fatigue, and improve immune function.
- **Magnesium.** Include nuts, seeds, and avocados to relax muscles and support cellular energy production.
- **Omega-3.** Eat fatty fish, chia seeds, or walnuts to reduce inflammation and enhance brain function.
- **CoQ10.** Found in organ meats and supplementation, this supports mitochondrial energy production.

Energy Detox to Combat Fatigue

Ever wonder how children can play all day without needing food? It's because they're fully immersed in the joy of what they're doing. For this energy detox, I encourage you to reflect on the activities that make you lose track of time and prioritize doing them more often. By reconnecting with your inner child, you can rediscover a natural, effortless energy that fuels you from within.

Fatigue can feel overwhelming, but restoring your energy requires a combination of adding positive, uplifting habits and removing draining influences from your life. Try these energy-boosting habits and eliminate energy-draining activities to feel a new level of vitality and natural energy without boosters like caffeine. This nine-week energy detox plan will help you thrive and glow like a superstar while following the Foodie Diet, the ultimate guide to reclaiming your energy and living your best life.

It's time to let go of what drains you and embrace practices that restore, empower, and inspire you!

Here's a curated list to help you thrive and glow like a superstar.

Energy-Boosting Practices to *Add*:

- **Music.** Uplifting tunes can instantly boost your mood and energy.
- **Dancing.** Move your body freely. Dance is a joyful way to energize and release stress. I recommend taking dance breaks throughout the day.
- **Nature.** Spend time outdoors to reconnect with the natural world and recharge.
- **Rest.** Embrace quality downtime as a vital part of restoring your energy reserves.
- **Meditation.** A few minutes of mindfulness daily can help calm your mind and focus your energy.
- **Sunshine.** Natural sunlight supports vitamin D production and boosts your mood.
- **Positive thoughts.** Shift your mindset to focus on optimism and opportunities.
- **Gratitude.** Daily reflections on what you're thankful for can enhance your emotional resilience.

- **Breathwork.** Controlled breathing exercises increase oxygen flow and calm the nervous system.
- **Organizing spaces.** Declutter and create order to bring clarity and reduce mental fatigue. Donate and get rid of things that don't bring joy anymore!
- **Sleep.** Prioritize consistent, high-quality, restorative sleep to fuel your body and mind.
- **Studying new skills.** Engage in learning to stimulate your brain and break monotony. Finally, do what you've always wanted to try! Golf, diving, French cooking, or belly dancing?

Energy Drainers to *Avoid*:

- **Focusing on the past.** Let go of regret and focus on what you can control today.
- **Irregular sleep patterns.** Poor sleep disrupts your energy cycles, so stick to a regular schedule.
- **Chaos and messy places.** A cluttered environment can lead to a cluttered mind.
- **Being inactive/sedentary.** Regular movement is essential to sustain energy levels.
- **Social media scrolling.** Mindless scrolling drains time and mental energy, and comparison to others increases stress and fatigue.
- **Resentment and negative thoughts.** These weigh heavily on your emotional well-being.
- **24/7 news reading.** While paying attention to current events and being an informed citizen are important, constant exposure to the news, which often focuses on sensational events, can increase emotional stress.
- **Stress, fears, and anxiety.** Address these with mindfulness, therapy, or professional support.

Reverse Autoimmune Disorders with Food

Autoimmune conditions occur when the immune system mistakenly attacks the body's own tissues, perceiving them as threats. This leads to chronic inflammation and damage to specific organs or systems. Examples include rheumatoid arthritis, where the immune system targets joints; type 1 diabetes, which affects insulin-producing cells in the pancreas; Hashimoto's thyroiditis, an attack on the thyroid gland; and celiac disease, where gluten triggers an immune response that damages the small intestine. These conditions often have genetic, environmental, and lifestyle triggers.

Autoimmune disorders often stem from a combination of genetic predisposition, environmental triggers, and imbalances in the gut microbiome. I've helped many clients heal these conditions with nutrition education, new food habits, and dietary changes that I detailed in Chapter 5, in addition to advanced immune support, which can play a transformative role in managing and even reversing autoimmune conditions.

One of my favorite strategies is incorporating colostrum and mushroom complexes into a client's regimen. Colostrum, the nutrient-dense pre-milk fluid produced by mammals, is rich in antibodies, growth factors, and immune-supporting nutrients. It has been shown to strengthen the gut lining, reduce inflammation, and support overall immune regulation. Also for immune modulation is a product I've been using for many years and often recommend to my clients. Host Defense MyCommunity is a comprehensive mushroom complex featuring seventeen mushroom species, including lion's mane, reishi, chaga, cordyceps, and turkey tail. This liquid extract (or in supplement capsule form) is specifically designed to support immune health and is easy to incorporate into daily routines.

Mushrooms like lion's mane support cognitive function while beta-glucans from reishi and turkey tail have been shown to modulate immune function through specific receptor pathways and are renowned for their anti-inflammatory and immune-balancing properties. Together, these mushrooms create a potent synergy that promotes resilience and gut-immune health.

In terms of diet for autoimmune conditions, I recommend a paleo-style approach focused on nutrient-dense whole foods, which eliminates common triggers such as gluten, dairy, and processed sugars while emphasizing anti-inflammatory, whole, real, and microbiome-supportive foods. Chapter 5 outlines all of the nutrient-dense foods to increase in your diet.

The Histamine Issue

High histamine can manifest as fatigue, headaches, flushing, nasal congestion, skin issues, and digestive discomfort. One of my clients, Ken, a forty-two-year-old athlete from Paris, was disciplined in his training and diet yet struggled with persistent fatigue, slow recovery, and premature signs of aging like fine lines and dull skin. Despite eating a clean, nutrient-rich diet and maintaining peak physical fitness, he felt drained and frustrated, unable to pinpoint the cause of his low energy. Upon reviewing his food habits, we discovered his diet was rich in high-histamine foods like aged cheeses, fermented products, and spinach. After implementing a low-histamine diet and supplementing with diamine oxidase, Ken experienced significant improvements within weeks. His energy returned, recovery times shortened, and his skin regained its vibrancy. This highlighted how even healthy habits must align with individual biochemistry for optimal results.

Histamine is a chemical found naturally in every cell in our body, an important component of the immune and nervous systems. In addition to the histamine our body makes, it is also naturally present (or can develop) in certain foods. Histamine content is especially high in fermented foods. But wait—aren't fermented foods supposed to be good for you? Keep reading for an answer to that question.

Histamine Intolerance

- Histamine intolerance (HIT) isn't a true allergy like we see with bee stings or peanuts. HIT is a mismatch between too much histamine in the body and the speed at which the body clears it. If too much histamine is released, it is not broken down fast enough; a person doesn't feel well.
- Individual histamine tolerance varies from person to person. Picture histamine tolerance like a unique water bucket for each person, influenced by various health factors. As the bucket fills, symptoms may arise when it overflows. Notably, gut health plays a significant role in determining how your body responds to foods containing histamine. Understanding and managing your histamine tolerance is crucial for maintaining well-being.

Histamine can trigger the immune system and cause symptoms like swelling, rashes, and watery eyes. If it affects the nervous system, it may cause problems such as headaches, digestive problems, and pain.

Low-Histamine Diet: What to Avoid

The low-histamine diet is being used to treat problems such as rashes, headaches, bloating, and HIT. If you're dealing with HIT, certain foods that are normally considered healthy can actually make things worse. Here's what to avoid:

- **Fish.** Stay away from frozen, salted, or canned fish like sardines and tuna.
- **Milk and dairy.** Avoid fermented dairy products such as aged cheese, yogurt, sour cream, buttermilk, and kefir.
- **Probiotic-rich foods.** Skip fermented vegetables like sauerkraut, kimchi, and pickles, as well as fermented soy products like tempeh, miso, soy sauce, and natto. Even fermented grains, like sourdough bread, and condiments containing vinegar or ketchup made with tomatoes should be avoided.
- **Alcohol.** Watch out for wine, beer, champagne, and other alcoholic beverages—they're high in histamine.

Fermented foods are usually great for gut health, but when HIT is in the picture, they can be problematic. Focus on fresh, nonfermented foods to keep your symptoms in check.

Eat for Healthy Hair, Skin, and Nails

Nutrient deficiencies from restrictive diets and stress are often the root causes of hair loss and skin issues. Here's how I help my clients directly support the integrity of connective tissues, including strong, radiant hair, nails, and skin with a focus on nutrient-dense foods.

Hair health relies on specific amino acids like cysteine and proline, which are essential for keratin production, as well as proteins and micronutrients such as biotin, zinc, and iron that promote growth and resilience. Additionally, vitamin C and collagen peptides play a critical role in maintaining the structural integrity of connective tissues by supporting collagen synthesis, essential for healthy skin and hair follicles. These nutrients work synergistically to enhance the strength, elasticity, and glow of the skin and connective tissues.

Here's my approach and the science behind each choice:

- **Whole chicken and broth (monthly).** I use a whole chicken, including skin and organ meats like liver, heart, and gizzards, to make a collagen-rich broth. Organ meats provide high concentrations of vitamin A, iron, and B_{12}—essential for oxygenating hair follicles, boosting scalp moisture, and preventing hair loss.
- **Eggs during luteal phase.** Eggs are rich in biotin, choline, and vitamin D. Biotin fortifies the hair shaft while vitamin D activates new hair follicles. During the luteal phase, these nutrients help stabilize hormone levels, promoting stronger, thicker hair.
- **Fish.** Eat fish with the skin on for an added boost of collagen, which supports skin elasticity and hair strength, and omega-3 fatty acids, which reduce inflammation, nourish hair follicles, and enhance the skin's lipid barrier for improved hydration.
- **Goat cheese and yogurt.** Goat dairy is easier to digest than dairy from cows and offers probiotics for gut health, enhancing nutrient uptake. High in B_6 and B_{12}, these foods aid in cell renewal and hair growth by supporting protein synthesis.
- **Daily leafy greens.** I include arugula, kale, and Swiss chard for liver support and detoxification. These greens are packed with folate and iron, which boost scalp blood flow and deliver vital nutrients directly to hair roots.
- **Organ meats (monthly).** Liver, heart, sweetbreads, and kidneys provide bioavailable iron, zinc, vitamin A, and CoQ_{10}. Iron supports red blood cells, zinc strengthens follicles, vitamin A regulates scalp oil production, and Q_{10}

enhances cellular energy for hair regeneration. The science behind organ meat consumption is particularly compelling. Research shows that just one 4-ounce serving provides 731 percent of your daily vitamin A and 988 percent of vitamin B_{12}, essential for cell turnover and sebum production.

- **Flax seeds and psyllium husk.** I add these to my smoothies for omega-3s and fiber. Omega-3s reduce scalp inflammation and enhance hair density. Psyllium husk improves digestion and cholesterol levels, promoting efficient blood flow to hair roots. (You'll find a smoothie recipes in Chapter 9.)
- **Brazil nuts.** These nuts offer selenium, which boosts hair growth and fights oxidative damage.
- **Niacin (vitamin B3).** Chicken and lentils offer niacin, which increases scalp circulation, delivering oxygen and nutrients directly to follicles for robust growth.

The Dairy-Skin Connection: My Personal Journey

Learning about my body's dairy intolerance changed both my skin and my sleep. Like many of my clients, I spent years struggling with skin issues and snoring, never connecting these problems to what I was eating. After two surgeries for a deviated septum and having my tonsils removed—procedures that were supposed to solve my snoring—I was still waking up with a dry mouth in the morning. In addition to that, I struggled with skin issues—like hormonal acne and recurring rashes—and no amount of expensive creams or dermatologist visits could clear my skin either. Each doctor had a different solution, but none addressed the root cause!

The turning point came when I ran a food sensitivity test and committed to a twenty-one-day dairy detox. The results were remarkable—I was finally able to breathe through my nose and my skin began to clear. What I discovered through both personal experience and clinical research is that cow's milk proteins can trigger inflammatory responses that manifest in ways we don't usually associate with dairy: mucus formation, skin acne, and even respiratory issues.

A study published in the *Journal of Clinical Medicine* demonstrates how A1 casein (the protein found in cow's milk) can trigger inflammatory responses different from A2 casein found in goat and sheep milk.

This is why I now exclusively choose goat and sheep milk products. Our bodies process goat and sheep milk protein differently than they do cow's milk protein, and they're less likely to trigger inflammatory responses. I still get to enjoy my beloved cheeses—just from different sources. My favorites include fresh chèvre and aged pecorino, which provide all the pleasure of dairy without the inflammatory response.

Pro Tip from a Dietitian

If you're struggling with unexplained skin issues or chronic congestion, try the twenty-one-day dairy elimination protocol I described in Chapter 4 on bio-individuality and food sensitivities. Document your symptoms before and after. You might be surprised by improvements in areas you never connected to dairy sensitivity. Before you completely eliminate all dairy products, I highly recommend trying sheep and goat milk yogurt and kefir, as well as A2 cow's milk products, for their highly beneficial probiotics, healthy fats, and high-quality protein.

Feed Your Vision

I've struggled with eye health since I was ten years old and diagnosed with progressive myopia. Here's what I have learned and love recommending to my clients for supporting eye health.

I emphasize the importance of incorporating specific nutrients and foods to support eye health and sharper vision. In addition to anti-inflammatory foods, I love recommending options like blueberry-carrot juice, raw carrots as a snack, and my Waist-Slimming Red Cabbage Salad (featured in Chapter 9) that includes shredded carrots for a nutrient boost.

Carrots are rich in beta-carotene, a precursor to vitamin A, which is essential for maintaining healthy vision and supporting phototransduction—the process by which light is converted into signals in the retina. Blueberries are packed with anthocyanins, powerful antioxidants that help improve blood flow to the eyes and reduce oxidative stress, protecting against age-related vision decline.

Other key nutrients for eye health include

- **Lutein and zeaxanthin.** Found in leafy greens like kale and spinach, these carotenoids protect the retina and may reduce the risk of macular degeneration.
- **Astaxanthin.** This potent antioxidant found in seafood, like shrimp and salmon, supports ocular blood flow and overall eye function.

- **Vitamin C and E, zinc, and copper.** These nutrients work together to combat oxidative stress and slow the progression of age-related macular degeneration.

By incorporating these foods and nutrients into your daily diet, you can support your vision naturally while also benefiting your gut and overall health. Simple additions like a raw carrot snack at least once a week or a vibrant carrot juice (find carrot recipes in Chapter 9) nourish your body and also support long-term eye health.

GI Disorders

For individuals with GI disorders such as constipation, bloating, irritable bowel syndrome IBS, colitis, or Crohn's disease, diet must be approached with precision to target underlying inflammation, gut dysbiosis, and impaired digestion. In many cases, collaboration with a gastroenterologist is essential to ensure proper diagnosis, treatment, and long-term management. In addition to the anti-inflammatory foods outlined in Chapter 5, these strategies target the root causes of GI disorders and provide an opportunity to restore gut health while minimizing symptoms.

Pro Tip from a Dietitian

For all GI conditions, probiotics and prebiotics should be tailored to individual tolerance. Spore-based probiotics may be better tolerated by people with Crohn's while fermented foods like kimchi or sauerkraut can benefit those with IBS when introduced gradually.

Constipation

- Focus on soluble and insoluble fibers from foods like ground flaxseeds, chia seeds, and steamed leafy greens to regulate bowel movements without irritating the gut.
- Add magnesium-rich foods, such as pumpkin seeds and dark chocolate, or supplement with magnesium citrate for gentle stool softening.
- Incorporate Swedish bitters for enzymatic sufficiency. Sometimes, even taking enzymes can also help prioritize hydration by pairing water intake with electrolytes, such as coconut water or a pinch of sea salt, to help gut motility.

Bloating and IBS

- Implement a low-FODMAP (fermentable oligosaccharides, disaccharides, monosaccharides, and polyols) diet to identify and eliminate trigger foods, such as onions, garlic, and certain legumes, which ferment in the gut and exacerbate bloating.
- Include carminative herbs like fennel, peppermint, and ginger to soothe the digestive tract and reduce gas.
- Add digestive enzymes, particularly those with lactase and amylase, to support the breakdown of complex carbohydrates and lactose.
- I highly recommend doing a comprehensive stool test to check for bacterial overgrowth and dysbiosis. Once diagnosed, these conditions can be targeted with specific probiotic strains to alleviate symptoms.

Crohn's Disease

- Emphasize omega-3-rich foods, such as wild-caught salmon and sardines, to reduce intestinal inflammation and support mucosal healing.
- Integrate bone broth and collagen peptides to repair intestinal permeability and enhance gut lining integrity.
- Opt for nutrient-dense, easily digestible foods like cooked root vegetables, white rice, and lean proteins to minimize irritation during flare-ups.

Dietitian-Approved Gut Health Hacks

I have some easy, science-backed tips for you. These small changes can make a huge difference!

- Try salmon jerky as a protein-packed snack. Omega-3s in salmon are known to reduce inflammation and support gut health.
- Add superfood herbs like turmeric, which has powerful anti-inflammatory properties; ginger, which supports digestion; and mint, which helps soothe the digestive tract and reduce bloating. Incorporating these herbs into your meals can naturally support a healthier gut. I love ordering fresh mint tea at restaurants—especially since most don't offer much beyond green, black, or flavored teas. I simply ask for fresh mint from the bar, which many restaurants have on hand for mojitos, and request it with hot water. It's a simple, soothing digestive ritual.
- Don't underestimate the power of deep breathing! A few deep breaths before eating activate the vagus nerve,

which signals your body to enter rest-and-digest mode, improving digestion and nutrient absorption.

Herbal Support for Gut Lining Repair

Mucosal lining–restoring herbs are recommended when there is evidence of damage or irritation to the gut lining, often seen in conditions such as leaky gut syndrome, Crohn's disease, ulcerative colitis, gastritis, or IBS. These herbs help rebuild the protective barrier of the digestive tract, reduce inflammation, and support overall gut integrity.

1. **Chronic GI symptoms.** Persistent symptoms like bloating, diarrhea, constipation, or abdominal pain suggest possible gut-lining damage.
2. **Autoimmune conditions.** Disorders like Crohn's, ulcerative colitis, or celiac disease often involve gut-lining damage that can benefit from herbs like slippery elm or marshmallow root.
3. **Post-antibiotic use.** After antibiotics, gut mucosa may need support to recover from disruption to beneficial bacteria.
4. **Food sensitivities.** Individuals with multiple food sensitivities may have increased intestinal permeability—leaky gut—requiring mucosal repair.
5. **Acid reflux or gastritis.** Herbs can soothe irritation caused by excess stomach acid or inflammation of the gastric mucosa.
6. **Prolonged stress.** Chronic stress can weaken the gut barrier, making mucosal-rcstoring herbs helpful in rebuilding resilience.

My Favorite Herbs for Gut Health

These herbs can be enjoyed as soothing teas to support gut health, especially after periods of stress. My favorite is licorice tea, such as Traditional Medicinals Organic Licorice Root Tea, which helps repair the gut lining and reduce inflammation. For a calming option, try Heather's Tummy Teas Organic Slippery Elm Tea, which coats and soothes the digestive tract, or Alvita Organic Marshmallow Root Tea, known for its protective effects on mucosal tissues.

- **Slippery elm.** Coats and soothes the gut lining, reducing inflammation and irritation.
- **Marshmallow root.** Forms a protective layer over the mucosa, aiding in healing and reducing discomfort.
- **Deglycyrrhizinated licorice.** Supports mucosal repair and is particularly effective for acid reflux and gastritis.
- **Aloe vera.** Soothes irritation and promotes tissue repair, especially in inflammatory conditions.

Female Health: Connection Between Gut Microbiome and Candida, PCOS

I've seen how intimately gut health connects to conditions like PCOS (polycystic ovary syndrome, a common hormonal disorder in women of childbearing age) and recurring infections. Let me share how these seemingly separate issues often share a common root in gut health.

When clients come to me with PCOS symptoms or recurring candida infections, we start by addressing their gut microbiome.

Many women don't realize that frequent yeast infections and antibiotic use can trigger a cascade of issues, leading to food sensitivities and even affecting hormonal conditions like PCOS.

Here's my clinical approach to candida overgrowth, refined through years of working with female clients: Focus on foods that create an inhospitable environment for candida while supporting healthy gut microbiome balance. Following are my go-to alkaline recommendations that play a specific role in creating an environment where candida can't thrive:

- Bitter greens like arugula, watercress, and bok choy
- Sulfur-rich vegetables like scallions and fennel
- Antioxidant powerhouses like frozen cranberries and blueberries
- Blood sugar stabilizers like avocados, ghee, and fatty fish
- Clean proteins to support hormonal health, like grass-fed steak

Beyond diet, lifestyle changes are crucial. I guide my clients to

- Choose breathable cotton and linen clothing.
- Switch to organic skincare products.
- Support their bodies during and after antibiotic use.

Probiotic foods become your allies in this journey. I'm not talking about just any fermented foods—specifically, incorporate raw sauerkraut, kimchi, kombucha, and traditionally prepared sourdough. These foods help restore beneficial bacteria that keep candida in check.

For stubborn cases, I often recommend a high-dose probiotic supplement and undecylenic acid, a fatty acid that's shown remarkable results in my practice for maintaining healthy gut flora. This becomes particularly important for clients who've been on oral contraceptives or multiple rounds of antibiotics or have persistent, recurring candida infections.

Pro Tip from a Dietitian

Healing goes beyond just what you eat. Switch to breathable cotton and linen clothing, and use only organic personal care products. I recommend Dr. Bronner's products to my clients for their pure ingredients that support your body's natural pH balance.

You'll find detailed recipes in Chapter 9, including my Green Goddess Smoothie and Gut-Healing recipes, that are therapeutic tools designed to support both gut and female health.

Your Antiaging Arsenal: Essential Nutrients for Cellular Health

Let me share specific nutrient powerhouses that I recommend to my clients for optimal aging, focusing on compounds that directly support cellular function and repair.

Glutathione: Your Master Antioxidant

While you can't effectively absorb glutathione directly from supplements, you can boost your body's production through specific foods.

- Duck eggs contain two and a half times more selenium than chicken eggs, making them superior for glutathione synthesis.

- Brazil nuts are another powerhouse—just two nuts provide 100 percent of your daily selenium needs.
- Most fascinating is asparagus; six spears contain unique compounds that boost glutathione production by 650 percent.

Magnesium's Hidden Sources

Beyond the well-known sources, I guide my clients to unexpected magnesium richness in black sapote (150 mg per fruit), molasses (242 mg per tablespoon), and amaranth (160 mg per cooked cup). The magnesium in these foods is bound to specific organic compounds that show 96 percent higher absorption rates than supplemental forms.

Brain-Building Nutrients

- For choline, I recommend less obvious sources: sunflower lecithin (the most concentrated source, with 2,200 mg per tablespoon), quail eggs (50 percent more choline than chicken eggs), and purslane (a wild green with the highest choline content of any vegetable).
- CoQ_{10} appears naturally in the highest concentrations in reindeer heart (156mg/100g), followed by sardines (the only fish with significant levels at 64mg/100g). For plant sources, pistachios contain a unique form that's 300 percent more bioavailable than other nuts.
- Alpha-lipoic acid reaches therapeutic levels in organic potato skins, particularly purple varieties, which contain three to four times more alpha-lipoic acid than regular potatoes. Beet greens (not the roots) are another surprising source, especially when lightly steamed.

Pro Tip from a Dietitian

Combine these foods strategically—potato skin with sardines, or purslane in a pistachio pesto—to create synergistic nutrient absorption.

Creatine is one of the most well-researched and effective supplements I recommend for clients seeking advanced nutrition strategies to enhance performance and recovery, particularly for athletes. Known for its ability to increase phosphocreatine stores, creatine improves muscle strength and power during high-intensity exercise while supporting muscle growth through enhanced protein synthesis and cellular hydration. Beyond its athletic benefits, creatine plays a critical role in cognitive health by replenishing energy in brain cells, improving memory, and potentially protecting against neurodegenerative conditions like Parkinson's disease. It also aids recovery by reducing muscle damage and inflammation after intense workouts, speeding up the healing process. For older adults, creatine is invaluable for combating age-related muscle loss (sarcopenia) and maintaining physical strength, especially when paired with resistance training. With its proven ability to boost energy, improve recovery, and support both brain and muscle function, creatine is a cornerstone supplement for anyone focused on optimizing health and performance.

BCAAs and amino acid complexes are essential tools in advanced nutrition, particularly for individuals aiming to optimize muscle recovery, energy production, and overall metabolic health. The BCAAs—leucine, isoleucine, and valine—are unique in their ability to bypass liver metabolism and be directly used by muscles for energy during exercise. Leucine, in particular, triggers muscle protein synthesis, making BCAAs invaluable for preserving lean muscle mass and accelerating recovery after intense physical activity. Amino acid complexes, which contain all nine essential amino acids (EAAs), go a step further by providing the full spectrum of building blocks needed for protein repair and synthesis, supporting tissue health, enzyme function, and immune system resilience. Together, BCAAs and EAAs work synergistically to reduce muscle breakdown, enhance endurance, and improve overall recovery, making them ideal for athletes, active individuals, or anyone looking to maintain muscle mass while dieting or aging. These supplements are foundational for advanced nutritional strategies that target both performance and longevity.

Nature's Longevity Compounds: Beyond Basic Antioxidants

Let me share what excites me most about these sophisticated cellular supporters. They aren't just antioxidants; they're genetic modulators and cellular architects that can transform how we age.

Cellular Activators

Resveratrol fascinates me because it doesn't just fight free radicals—it actually speaks to your DNA through sirtuin activation. While many know it from red wine, I guide my clients to more concentrated sources. For example, organic muscadine grapes contain forty times more resveratrol than regular grapes, and Japanese knotweed extract provides the highest concentration found in nature.

Quercetin's power lies in its dual action—it's both a senolytic (removing aged cells) and a natural antihistamine. Red onions contain the highest concentration (quercetin becomes more bioavailable when onions are lightly sautéed) while capers pack 180 mg per 100 g—the highest food concentration known.

Cellular Energy and Cleanup

NAD+ levels decline 50 percent every twenty years after age forty, making NAD precursors crucial. What's fascinating is how specific foods can boost NAD+ production: Wild salmon roe contains 300 percent more NAD+ precursors than muscle meat while sun-exposed mushrooms show significantly higher levels due to their unique ability to convert UV light into NAD+ building blocks.

Medicinal Mushrooms and Shilajit: Ancient Wisdom Meets Modern Science

Each medicinal mushroom offers unique neurotrophic compounds. Lion's mane contains erinacines and hericenones that cross the blood-brain barrier to stimulate nerve growth factor production. Clinical studies show that 3 g daily improves cognitive scores. Shilajit, a complex of over eighty-four minerals, interests me particularly for its fulvic acid content and ability to enhance mitochondrial energy production. I recommend it with coffee or tea first thing in the morning.

Inflammation and Aging

As we've learned, inflammation is at the root of most diseases—and it also plays a key role in weight imbalance, whether it's unexplained weight gain or difficulty losing weight, as well as in the aging process. For health and longevity, lowering inflammation is key. Add broccoli, spinach, bok choy, asparagus, celery, kale, Swiss chard, and zucchini to your meals, either in salads, stir-fries, or as a side to your main dishes.

Here's a tip: Create an antioxidant plate by combining various food sources. For example, pair your wild salmon with steamed broccoli, add caramelized red onions, and finish with a handful of blueberries for dessert. This isn't just a delicious meal—it's a powerful antiaging protocol working at the cellular level.

The Foodie's Guide to Advanced Nutrition: Where Joy Meets Longevity

Let me bring together everything we've discussed to this point and show you why the Foodie Diet isn't just another eating plan but a sophisticated approach to extending your health span while savoring every bite. In my practice, I've seen how combining the joy of eating with strategic nutrient optimization creates something remarkable: sustainable health that doesn't feel like a sacrifice.

Remember, the goal isn't to turn every meal into a scientific equation. It's about understanding how to incorporate these powerful nutrients into meals you genuinely enjoy. Whether it's starting your day with NAC-rich eggs, adding taurine-packed seafood to your lunch, or enjoying an alpha-lipoic acid boost from dinner's greens, every bite can work double duty for taste and longevity. When you understand how to pair your favorite foods with longevity-boosting compounds like NAD+, CoQ_{10}, and glutathione, every meal becomes an opportunity for cellular renewal.

In the end, the Foodie Diet proves what I've always believed: The most effective diet for longevity is one that brings you joy while nourishing your cells. What good is a long life if you can't enjoy your food along the way?

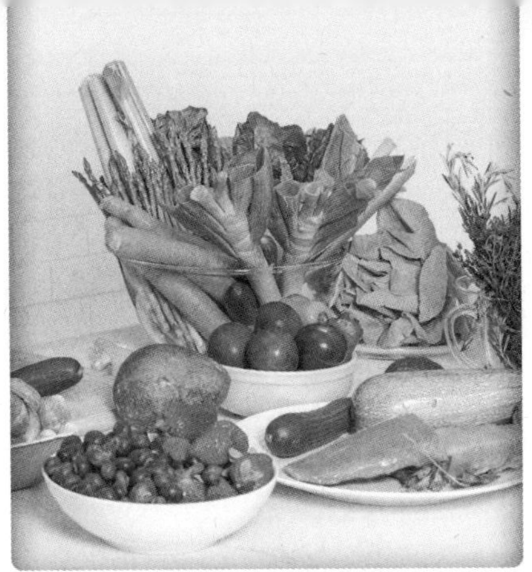

Chapter 9
Foodie Kitchen Essentials, Food Shopping List, and Recipes

The kitchen is where health transformation really happens. Not in fancy supplements or complicated protocols, but in simple, deliberate acts of combining high-quality ingredients into nourishing meals. This chapter isn't just about recipes—it's about empowering you to discover new food combinations and create meals that serve both your body metabolism and your soul. Or, as I like to say, "Bring sexy back into the kitchen!" And by sexy, I mean excitement, vitality, and high-vibrational energy. It's so much fun to cook with your loved ones while enjoying food that tastes amazing and makes you feel your best.

When I cook, I follow one simple rule: Maximize nutrient density while minimizing complexity. Here are my go-to recipes from my *Cooking for High Performers* cookbook, which I used to give to my clients at the end of the consultation to follow this principle. These aren't just recipes; they're formulas for optimal healthy and physical performance, derived from my childhood and cooking for my family, and perfected through years of working with clients who need real solutions for their busy lives.

Quality Ingredients

Your meals are only as good as your ingredients, and science shows us why. Grass fed meats contain significantly higher levels of anti-inflammatory omega-3 fatty acids compared to conventional meat, while wild-caught fish provide pure forms of DHA and EPA without the contamination risks of farmed varieties. Pasture-raised eggs deliver twice the vitamin E and omega-3s of conventional eggs, making them a superior choice for brain and heart health.

When it comes to produce, I recommend shopping at farmers' markets for local and seasonal vegetables and fruits containing peak nutrients because they're harvested at optimal ripeness. I always tell my clients to get to know their farmers—look at their hands, look into their eyes, and talk to them. Ask questions, especially if you don't recognize what they're selling; it could be seasonal vegetables like rapini or raab. Don't hesitate to ask them for recipe inspiration for the seasonal foods they're offering! Choosing organic options, particularly for the Environmental Working Group's Dirty Dozen, helps minimize exposure to pesticides that can disrupt our endocrine system and gut microbiome.

No-Waste Policy

In nature, nothing goes to waste, and this philosophy can transform how we cook and eat. I recommend embracing nose-to-tail eating, especially with organic, farm-raised meats, by including nutrient-dense organ meats like tongue, heart, liver, and sweetbreads. I also make the most of vegetables: Stems of cilantro go into dips; broccoli stems add flavor and fiber to bone or vegetable broths; and I even use lemons in smoothies by trimming off the yellow peel to remove bitterness while keeping the nutrient-rich white pith. These small choices reduce waste and maximize nutrition.

When it comes to dining out, the perspective of Suze Orman, America's favorite personal finance expert, is worth considering: "I refuse to eat out. I think that eating out on any level is one of the biggest wastes of money out there." Cooking at home not only saves money but also allows you to use every part of your ingredients efficiently—creating meals that are both nutritious and sustainable. Plus, there's a deep satisfaction in preparing something with your own hands; it can be fun, creative, and even relaxing when you make the time for it.

Kitchen Equipment

Some of these items are expensive, but they often outlast their less pricey counterparts, making them a better investment in the long run for both your wallet and the environment. Here are the essentials I use most in my kitchen:

- **Stainless-steel or cast-iron pots and pans.** These are the only two types of cookware in my kitchen. I avoid other materials due to potential health risks or lack of durability.
- **Immersion blender and food processor.** An immersion blender is one of my favorite kitchen tools! It's perfect for

making soups and dips when a full-size blender feels like overkill.

- **Vitamix blender.** This is a fantastic investment and worth every penny! Over the last decade, I've owned two, upgrading only for size. Vitamix blenders last forever and are unparalleled for making the smoothest smoothies, nut milks, blended soups, and hummus.
- **Mason jars and glass storage containers.** I rely heavily on glass storage for both the refrigerator and pantry. I use mason jars and glass storage containers to store prepped meals, dressings, cut vegetables, and leftovers. They're also perfect for pantry staples like grains, nuts, seeds, and dried fruit. I prefer glass because it's nontoxic, nonporous, and doesn't leach chemicals into food—especially when exposed to heat. In contrast, plastic containers can release harmful compounds like BPA and phthalates when heated, even at low temperatures. This is especially concerning when storing hot food or microwaving leftovers. Choosing glass is a simple but powerful upgrade that supports both your health and your long-term sustainability goals.
- **Parchment paper.** I use parchment paper instead of foil, as studies have shown that aluminum foil can leach aluminum into food when exposed to high heat. Parchment paper is perfect for roasting vegetables, steaming fish, or wrapping snacks and other food for on-the-go convenience.

The Science of Spices

I highly recommend investing in a good spice rack. This is the secret to transforming simple recipes and high-quality ingredients into dishes that taste amazing. The key lies in the spice mix—*it adds flavor without adding calories!*

The healing power of herbs and spices lies in their bioactive compounds. Turmeric's active compound curcumin becomes 2,000 percent more bioavailable when combined with black pepper's piperine. Ginger contains gingerols that reduce inflammation and support digestion. Cinnamon's compounds help regulate insulin sensitivity, while fresh herbs provide concentrated sources of antioxidants that protect our cells from oxidative stress. Each recipe in this chapter harnesses these powerful ingredients in ways that both nourish your body and delight your senses. True healing happens when we combine scientific knowledge with the joy of cooking and eating.

When it comes to recipe inspiration, I admire these heroes for their incredible flavor combinations, simple yet impactful recipes, and commitment to promoting a farm-to-table lifestyle: chef and food activist Kimbal Musk, farmer Julius Roberts, cooking show host Daphne Oz, and supermodel Gisele Bündchen.

Most of the recipes featured in this chapter are those I made on various TV shows because of how quick and easy they are, and I often recommend them to my clients. In this chapter, you'll discover

- Quick and easy, nourishing dinner ideas with protein at every meal
- How to master a balanced salad for lunch to load up on polyphenols and antioxidants
- Hormone-balancing breakfasts
- Plant-based deliciousness to take advantage of high-fiber foods for gut health
- Gut-healing recipes
- Nutritious and delicious soups
- Nutrient-dense smoothies and drinks
- Low-sugar delectable desserts

My Dietitian-Approved Shopping List

The Foodie Diet prioritizes anti-inflammatory, nutrient-dense foods that support immunity, digestive health, metabolism, and overall well-being. Following is your go-to shopping list, meticulously curated. Use the shopping list when you visit the supermarket. Afterward, you'll also discover recipes to incorporate these foods into your meals. The key is to always ensure that your pantry and fridge are filled with healthy options because what you surround yourself with matters!

> If you surround yourself with healthy food,
> you will end up eating healthy food.

Vegetables. Focus on organic, non-GMO, farm-fresh options. These nutrient-packed vegetables should form the foundation of your meals:

- **Cruciferous vegetables.** Broccoli, kale, Swiss chard, broccolini, Brussels sprouts, cauliflower, cabbage (red, green, Napa, savoy)
- **Leafy greens.** Spinach, salad greens, arugula, mustard greens, dandelion greens, watercress
- **Root and stalk vegetables.** Radishes (daikon, red), celery, leeks, fennel, asparagus, bamboo shoots, jicama
- **Allium vegetables.** Onions, garlic, shallots, scallions, chives
- **Specialty greens.** Endive, radicchio, bok choy, cucumbers
- **Flavor enhancers.** Cilantro, dill, parsley
- **Peppers.** Bell peppers, shishito peppers, hot peppers
- **Other.** Artichokes, zucchini, sprouts, aloe vera

Fruits. Antioxidant-rich, low-glycemic fruits (fresh or frozen) are essential for immune and metabolic health. Choose among the following:

- **Berries.** Strawberries, raspberries, blueberries, blackberries, mulberries, sour cherries, gooseberries, sea buckthorn, goji berries, red and black currants
- **Citrus fruits.** Pomegranates, tangerines, oranges, pomelos
- **Tropical fruits.** Guava, mango, papaya
- **Stone fruits.** Apricots, plums, nectarines, peaches
- **Other.** Kiwi, figs, cantaloupe, watermelon, persimmons, grapes, pears, bananas

Protein and fats. Choose grass-fed, pasture-raised, and wild-caught options for optimal nutrition:

- **Seafood.** Salmon, salmon roe, mackerel, sardines, trout, shellfish (oysters, mussels)
- **Poultry.** Free-range chicken, turkey, duck
- **Meat.** Grass-fed beef, lamb, buffalo
- **Organ meats.** Chicken and beef livers
- **Eggs.** Cage-free, organic eggs
- **Plant-based proteins.** Lentils (yellow, red, green), edamame, miso, tofu, sprouted beans (adzuki, black beans, chickpeas/garbanzo)
- **Nuts and seeds.** Brazil nuts, walnuts, macadamia nuts, pistachios, almonds, baruka nuts, pecans, coconuts, cashews, pumpkin seeds, flaxseeds, chia seeds, hemp seeds, sesame seeds/tahini

Starchy vegetables and grains. Prioritize organic, non-GMO options:

- **Purple potatoes, yams, corn, mushrooms, butternut squash, Jerusalem artichoke**

- **Whole grains** such as quinoa, farro, and sprouted wheat
- **Specialty items.** For enhanced flavor and additional health benefits:
    - **Spices.** Ginger, turmeric, cinnamon
    - **Healthy oils.** Extra virgin olive oil, avocado oil, coconut oil, ghee
    - **Fermented foods.** Miso, kimchi, sauerkraut, pickles, fermented olives, beets

Breads and Crackers

- **Bread.** Locally made seven-grain bread or sourdough if eating gluten; gluten-free sourdough bread by Simple Kneads, grain-free bread by Base Culture
- **Crackers.** Gluten-free or grain-free crackers by Hu Kitchen or Simple Mills
- **Pizza crusts.** Grain-free, cauliflower-based, or organic gluten-free options

Dairy and Dairy Alternatives

- Coconut yogurt and ice cream by So Delicious
- A2-type organic milk from grass-fed sources
- Organic goat or sheep's milk cheese (soft/fresh and hard/aged)
- Goat's milk yogurt by Redwood Hill Farm (or sheep's milk)

Pantry essentials. Stock your pantry and refrigerator with items rich in polyphenols, antioxidants, and functional nutrients. Always choose quality organic products.

- Fruits and berries for smoothies, desserts, and water flavoring (cherries, açai)
- Vegetables for smoothies, stews, soups, and stir-fries

- Proteins: Grass-fed meat from Butcher Box, Force of Nature; wild Alaskan seafood and berries from Vital Choice, Northwest Wild Foods
- Organic grass-fed ghee (clarified butter)
- Plant-based milks: Almond, coconut, hemp, macadamia, cashew, sesame, pistachio
- Matcha and green tea
- Herbal teas: Echinacea, burdock root, elderberry, ginger, chaga tea, turmeric tea

Pasta and Grains

- Gluten-free quinoa or rice-based pasta
- High-protein options: Lentil, chickpea, bean-based pasta by Banza or Tolerant Foods
- Spaghetti squash pasta
- Gluten-free whole grains: Wild rice, cassava, sorghum, teff, amaranth, millet, brown rice

Herbs and spices. Fresh and dried options for enhanced flavor:

- Basil, rosemary, thyme, cilantro, parsley, dill, sage
- Italian herbs mix, zaatar, Herbs de Provence
- Turmeric, cinnamon, ginger, garlic, sea salt, red pepper flakes, chili powder

Sweeteners and Treats

- Honey in the comb
- Bee pollen
- Dark chocolate (70 percent cacao and higher)

Freezer Essentials

- Gluten-free whole grains

- Vegetables: Zucchini, peas, corn, mixed vegetables, spinach, artichoke hearts, bell peppers, pearl onions, fava beans
- Proteins: Wild-caught sardines (Vital Choice, Patagonia Provisions), salmon or beef jerky
- Fiber for smoothies: Psyllium husk, acacia fiber

Recipes

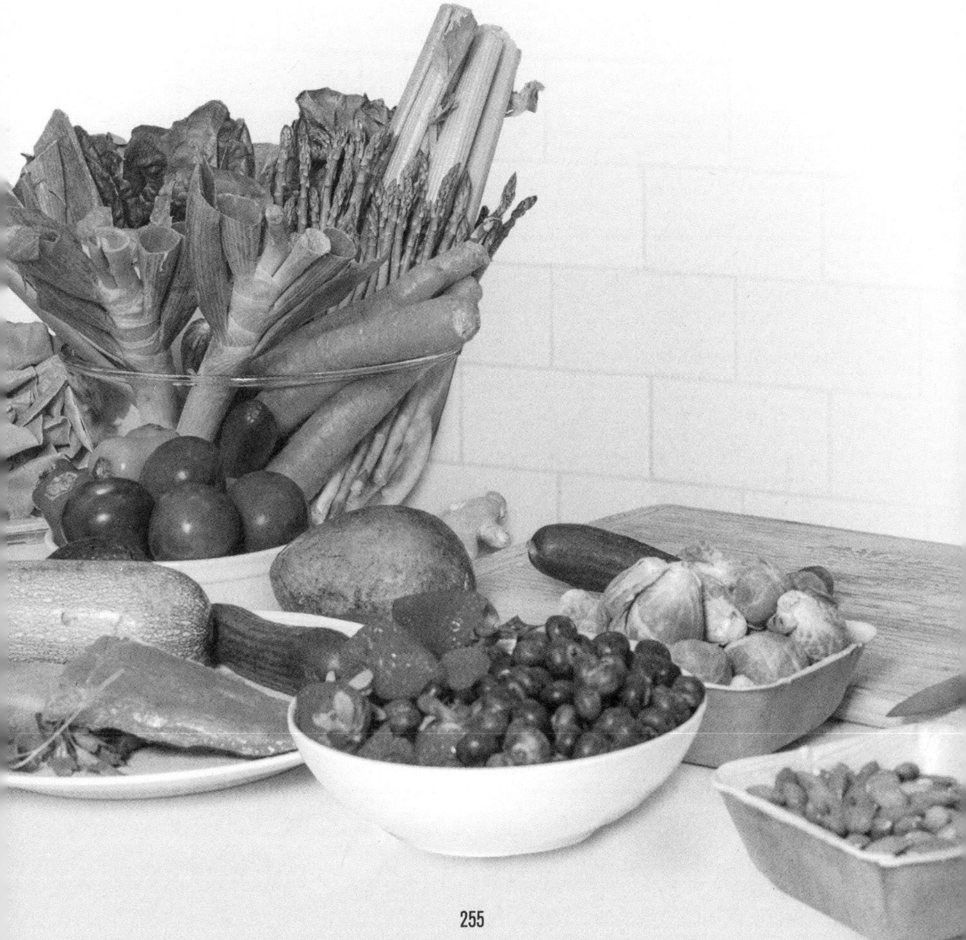

Quick and Nourishing Dinner Ideas

Here are my go-to recipes that combine brain-boosting nutrients with satisfying flavors—perfect for busy weeknights. Once you master these, there's absolutely no need to rely on food delivery apps. These simple, flavorful recipes truly showcase where functional food meets flavor:

ONE-PAN MEDITERRANEAN HERB SALMON

PREP TIME: 5 minutes
COOK TIME: 15 minutes
SERVES: 2

For the salmon:

1 bunch asparagus, woody ends trimmed

1 cup cherry tomatoes

4 tablespoons extra virgin olive oil

4 cloves garlic, minced

Sea salt and black pepper to taste

2 (6 oz.) wild-caught salmon fillets

1 lemon

Fresh herbs (dill, parsley, basil)

1. Preheat oven to 400°F. Line a baking sheet with parchment paper.
2. Arrange asparagus and tomatoes on one side of the pan. Drizzle with 2 tablespoons olive oil, add half the garlic, season with salt and pepper.
3. Place salmon fillets on the other side, skin-side down. Drizzle with remaining olive oil, add remaining garlic, squeeze half the lemon, and sprinkle with fresh herbs.
4. Roast for 12 to 15 minutes until salmon is just cooked through and vegetables are tender-crisp.
5. Serve with remaining lemon wedges.

PRO TIP: Choose salmon with bright color and firm flesh. The omega-3s in wild salmon combine with the antioxidants in vegetables to maximize nutrient absorption.

TURMERIC-GINGER CHICKEN BOWL

PREP TIME: 10 minutes
COOK TIME: 20 minutes
SERVES: 2

For the chicken:

2 organic chicken breasts

1 tablespoon turmeric

1 thumb fresh ginger, grated

2 cloves garlic, minced

Black pepper to taste

2 tablespoons coconut oil

For the bowl:

1 tablespoon ghee

1 head cauliflower, riced

2 cups mixed greens (kale, spinach, chard)

1. Season chicken with turmeric, grated ginger, garlic, and black pepper.
2. Heat coconut oil in a large skillet. Cook chicken for 6 to 7 minutes on each side until golden and cooked through.
3. In another pan, melt ghee, and add cauliflower rice. Cook for 5 to 7 minutes until tender.
4. Add greens to cauliflower rice, and cook until just wilted.
5. Slice chicken, and serve over cauliflower rice and greens.

PRO TIP: Adding black pepper increases turmeric absorption by 2,000 percent. This combination helps reduce inflammation while providing sustained energy.

GRASS-FED STEAK AND RAINBOW VEGETABLES

PREP TIME: 10 minutes
COOK TIME: 20 minutes
SERVES: 2

For the steak:

2 grass-fed rib eye or sirloin steaks

Sea salt and black pepper

2 tablespoons extra virgin olive oil

2 cloves garlic, crushed

Fresh rosemary and thyme

For the rainbow vegetables:

1 red bell pepper, sliced

2 carrots, rainbow if available

1 zucchini

1 cup Brussels sprouts, halved

2 tablespoons avocado oil

Sea salt and herbs to taste

1. Bring steaks to room temperature, season generously with salt and pepper.
2. Preheat the oven to 425°F. Toss vegetables with avocado oil and salt and herbs, and spread on a baking sheet.
3. Roast vegetables for 20 minutes until caramelized, stirring halfway.
4. Meanwhile, heat olive oil in a cast-iron skillet. Add crushed garlic and herbs.
5. Sear steaks for 4 to 5 minutes on each side for medium rare. Rest for 5 to 10 minutes before slicing.

PRO TIP: Iron absorption from grass-fed beef increases when paired with vitamin C–rich vegetables. This combination supports optimal energy and blood building.

FIVE-SPICE MISO COD

PREP TIME: 10 minutes (plus optional marinating)
COOK TIME: 15 minutes
SERVES: 2

2 tablespoons white miso paste

1 tablespoon mirin

1 teaspoon Chinese five-spice

2 (6 oz.) black cod or cod fillets

2 baby bok choy, halved

2 tablespoons coconut aminos

1-inch piece ginger, julienned

Sesame seeds for garnish

1. Mix miso, mirin, and five-spice. Spread on fish, marinate for 15 minutes to overnight.
2. Preheat oven to 400°F.
3. Place fish on a parchment-lined baking sheet, and bake for 12 to 15 minutes until flaky.
4. Meanwhile, steam bok choy for 3 to 4 minutes, and drizzle with coconut aminos.
5. Garnish with ginger and sesame seeds.

PRO TIP: Fermented miso provides probiotics while five-spice supports digestion. This meal combines gut health with protein for optimal absorption.

HEALTHY AND DELICIOUS MEATBALLS

These flavorful and nutrient-packed meatballs are a perfect combination of lean protein, vibrant vegetables, and aromatic herbs. Using lean ground beef or turkey as the base, this recipe is elevated by the addition of carrots, celery, and sweet onion, providing a burst of nutrients and natural sweetness. Pair with brown rice or whole-grain pasta for a wholesome meal that's as satisfying as it is nutritious.

PREP TIME: 20 minutes
COOK TIME: 45–60 minutes
SERVES: 6–8

2 pounds lean ground beef or turkey

1 large sweet onion, thinly sliced into rounds

3 carrots, grated

4 celery stalks, finely chopped

3 garlic cloves, minced or pressed

2 tablespoons olive oil

2 teaspoons dried oregano, thyme, and basil

½ teaspoon onion powder

1 teaspoon salt

½ teaspoon black pepper

2 (28 oz.) cans crushed organic tomatoes

1. Prepare the mixture. In a large bowl, combine the ground meat, onion, grated carrots, celery, garlic, olive oil, dried herbs, onion powder, salt, and pepper. Mix thoroughly until all ingredients are evenly incorporated.
2. Form the meatballs. Roll the mixture into balls of your preferred size and place them in a large skillet or baking dish.
3. Add tomatoes. Pour one can of crushed tomatoes over the meatballs, ensuring they are evenly coated. Add a sprinkle of additional herbs and garlic, if desired.
4. Bake. Preheat your oven to 375°F. Place the skillet or baking dish in the oven and bake uncovered for 45 to 60 minutes, until the meatballs are cooked through and slightly browned on the outside.
5. Serve. Serve the meatballs hot with brown rice or whole-grain pasta. For added flavor, drizzle with a little olive oil and sprinkle with fresh herbs or Parmesan cheese, if desired.

SAUTÉED BEEF LIVER WITH CARAMELIZED ONIONS

Beef liver is one of the most nutrient-dense foods you can eat, loaded with iron, vitamin A, and B vitamins. Paired with caramelized onions, this classic dish transforms the richness of liver into a flavorful and comforting meal.

PREP TIME: 10 minutes (optional 30 minutes soaking)
COOK TIME: 20 minutes
SERVES: 2–3

1 pound beef liver, sliced into thin strips

¼ cup flour (optional, for dusting)

2 tablespoons olive oil or ghee

2 large onions, thinly sliced

2 tablespoons butter (optional, for extra richness)

½ teaspoon salt

½ teaspoon black pepper

½ teaspoon smoked paprika (optional)

½ cup beef broth (optional, for a saucier dish)

Fresh parsley, chopped, for garnish

Prepare the liver:

- If desired, soak the liver in milk or water with a splash of lemon juice for 30 minutes to reduce its strong flavor. Drain and pat dry with a paper towel.

Optional: Lightly dust the liver slices with flour for a crispier texture.

Caramelize the onions:

- Heat olive oil in a large skillet over medium heat.
- Add the sliced onions and cook, stirring occasionally, for 10 to 15 minutes until they are soft and golden brown. Lower heat if they start to burn. Remove the onions from the skillet and set aside.

Cook the liver:

- In the same skillet, melt butter (if using) and heat over medium-high heat.
- Add the liver slices in a single layer and season with salt, pepper, and smoked paprika (if using). Cook for 2 to 3 minutes on each side until browned but still slightly pink in the center (overcooking can make liver tough).

Combine and serve:

- Return the caramelized onions to the skillet, stirring gently to combine with the liver. If a saucier dish is desired, deglaze the pan with beef broth and simmer for 1 to 2 minutes.
- Garnish with fresh parsley and serve immediately.

Serving suggestions: This dish pairs beautifully with mashed potatoes, cauliflower puree, or steamed green beans for a nutrient-packed, hearty meal. Whether you're a seasoned liver fan or trying it for the first time, the sweetness of the onions balances the richness of the liver perfectly!

CRUCIFEROUS VEGGIES FOR DINNER (AND LEFTOVERS FOR LUNCH)

Basic Greens for Any Occasion

This versatile recipe makes 3 servings (1 serving ≈ 1 cup). Add cooked vegetables to any base of leafy greens for a nutrient-packed side dish or salad topper.

PREP TIME: 5–10 minutes
COOK TIME: 10–15 minutes
SERVES: 3

1 large bunch of kale, collards, chard, or bok choy, washed

1 tablespoon olive oil or coconut oil

2–3 cloves garlic, minced or sliced into slivers

½ cup vegetable or chicken broth

Optional: Minced fresh ginger or your choice of herbs and spices

Additional Flavor Add-Ons

Take your greens or broccoli to the next level with these delicious additions:

Ghee

Smoked or truffle salt

Truffle hot sauce

"Everything but the Bagel" seasoning

1. For kale or collards, remove the tough center stem and chop or slice the leaves into small pieces. For chard or bok choy, simply chop into small pieces.
2. Heat olive oil in a large skillet over medium heat. Sauté the garlic for about 30 seconds until fragrant.
3. Add the chopped greens and sauté for 3 to 4 minutes. For chard or bok choy, this is sufficient. For kale or collards, add the broth, cover, and simmer over low heat for 10 minutes.
4. For seasoned greens, enhance the flavor with small amounts of dry chipotle pepper, balsamic vinegar, ground cumin, or curry powder.

Broccoli Side Dish

Bright green and full of nutrients, this broccoli dish is quick and easy to prepare.

PREP TIME: 5 minutes
COOK TIME: 10 minutes
SERVES: 3

Fresh broccoli, cut into florets

1 tablespoon olive oil or ghee

Salt and lemon to taste

1. Steam the broccoli in a pan with a little water until it turns bright green (for about 3 to 5 minutes).
2. Drain the water, then briefly sauté the broccoli in olive oil. Season with salt and a squeeze of fresh lemon juice.

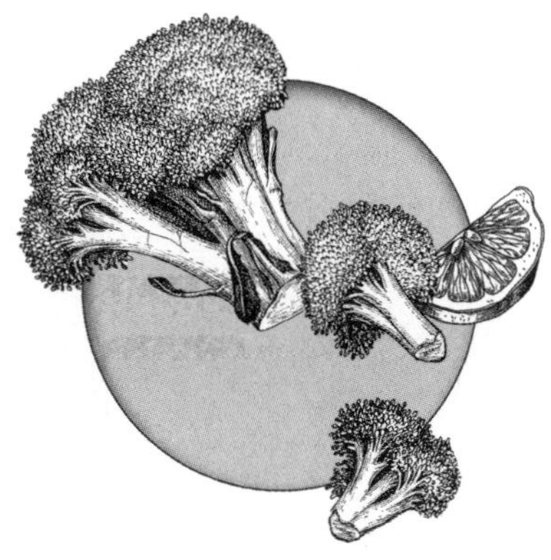

ROASTED CAULIFLOWER WITH PINE NUTS

PREP TIME: 10 minutes
COOK TIME: 25 minutes
SERVES: 3 (1 serving = about 1 cup)

1 head cauliflower, broken into florets

2 cloves garlic, peeled and minced

2 tablespoons extra virgin olive oil

1 teaspoon fresh rosemary, finely chopped

½ cup raw pine nuts

¼ teaspoon sea salt

¼ teaspoon freshly ground black pepper

Optional: ¼ teaspoon turmeric powder

1. Preheat your oven to 425°F.
2. In a large mixing bowl, combine the cauliflower florets and minced garlic. Drizzle with olive oil and toss to coat evenly.
3. Sprinkle the cauliflower with rosemary, pine nuts, salt, and pepper (add turmeric if desired). Mix thoroughly to ensure all pieces are evenly seasoned.
4. Spread the mixture evenly on a baking sheet in a single layer.
5. Roast, uncovered, for 20 to 25 minutes, or until the tops and edges of the cauliflower are lightly browned. Stir halfway through if needed to prevent over-browning.
6. Serve immediately.

PRO TIP: Pair this dish with your favorite protein for a complete meal, or serve it over a bed of leafy greens for a hearty salad.

PLANT-BASED DELICIOUSNESS: CROWD-PLEASING HOMEMADE HUMMUS

PREP TIME: 10 minutes
COOK TIME: 0 minutes
SERVES: 4

1 can of chickpeas (remove skins for creamier texture)

½ lemon, juiced

3 teaspoons tahini

Spices: salt, cumin, paprika, chili flakes

2 tablespoons extra virgin olive oil

Garnishes: sumac, pomegranate seeds, roasted chickpeas, thinly sliced radishes, and mint

Optional flavor additions:

- Roasted beets for a vibrant pink hue
- Roasted garlic for extra depth
- Roasted bell peppers for a smoky twist

1. In a food processor, combine the chickpeas with ½ cup of water. Add the lemon juice, tahini, and spices. Blend until creamy, adding more water as needed for desired consistency. Transfer to a serving bowl.
2. Garnish with olive oil, sumac, pomegranate seeds, roasted chickpeas, thinly sliced radishes, and mint.
3. Serve with pita chips, whole radishes, fennel, cucumbers, and carrots.

Preparing Dried Chickpeas (Optional):

1. Start the day before. In a medium bowl, cover dried chickpeas with 2 inches of water and stir in 1 teaspoon of baking soda. Refrigerate overnight.
2. Drain and rinse the chickpeas under cold water.
3. In a medium saucepan, cover the chickpeas with 2 inches of fresh water. Add another teaspoon of baking soda and bring to a boil. Simmer over moderate heat for about 1 hour, or until very tender.
4. Drain, reserving ½ cup of cooking water, and rinse under cold water.

The following are some variations of hummus that are versatile, vibrant, and sure to impress at any gathering:

GREEN HUMMUS

1. Blanch curly spinach in boiling salted water until wilted (about 10 seconds). Cool under running water and squeeze dry.
2. Using a blender, add the spinach and 1 cup of mixed herbs (parsley, cilantro, dill) to the basic hummus ingredients. Blend until smooth.
3. Garnish with olive oil, toasted pine nuts, chopped herbs, and kale chips. Serve with harissa for a spicy kick.

PINK HUMMUS

1. Wrap 3 medium beets first in foil, then in parchment paper on the outside. Roast at 425°F for 40 minutes, or until tender. Let cool, then peel and chop.
2. Add the roasted beets to the basic hummus ingredients and blend until smooth.
3. Garnish with toasted almonds, crumbled feta cheese, dukkah, sliced scallions, and watermelon radishes.

GREEN LENTILS WITH SPINACH AND PANCETTA

Green lentils are one of my go-to ingredients—they're packed with protein, full of fiber, and serve as a versatile base for all kinds of meals. Whether paired with sausages and mustardy aioli, pan-fried fish with salsa verde, or slow-roasted lamb and anchovy, they bring depth and balance to any dish.

In this recipe, I pair them with roasted pumpkin and goat cheese for a hearty, satisfying meal, but the beauty of lentils is in their adaptability. Leftovers can be repurposed into a pasta sauce with chili oil and Parmesan or transformed into a curried lentil soup—one of my family's classics.

PREP TIME: 20 minutes
COOK TIME: 45 minutes
SERVES: 6

1 large yellow onion

1 leek

2 carrots

3 celery stalks

4 tablespoons olive oil

5¼ ounces diced pancetta (optional)

Salt and pepper, to taste

1 generous glass of white wine

2½ cups green lentils

5 bay leaves

A few sprigs of fresh thyme

5 cups chicken stock, vegetable stock, or water

1 pound spinach

1 heaped tablespoon Dijon mustard

A big handful of fresh parsley, chopped

Optional Toppings:

- Roasted pumpkin or butternut squash: Toss chunks in olive oil and roast at 400°F for 35 to 40 minutes until caramelized and golden.
- Goat cheese, for dolloping

1. Prepare the vegetables. Finely dice the onion, leek, carrots, and celery.
2. Cook the base. Heat the olive oil in a large pot over medium heat. Add the diced vegetables and pancetta, if using, and season generously with salt and pepper. Sauté gently for 15 to 20 minutes, stirring occasionally, until the vegetables are soft and sweet.
3. Add the wine and lentils. Pour in the white wine, letting the alcohol cook off for a minute. Rinse the green lentils in a sieve, then add them to the pot. Stir well to coat.
4. Simmer the lentils. Add the bay leaves, thyme, and enough stock to just cover the lentils. Bring to a gentle simmer, then cook for about 30 minutes, stirring occasionally, until the lentils are tender but still have a slight bite.
5. Finish with spinach and mustard. Once the lentils are cooked, stir in the spinach and cook for 1 to 2 minutes, just until wilted. Remove from heat, then stir in the Dijon mustard and chopped parsley. Adjust seasoning with more salt, pepper, and mustard, if needed.
6. Serve. Plate the lentils with roasted pumpkin or squash, and top with dollops of goat cheese for extra creaminess.

Storage and Leftover Ideas: This dish keeps well in the fridge for up to 3 days. Leftovers are really versatile:

- Blend or mash them for a hearty pasta sauce with chili oil and Parmesan.
- Add a bit of water and curry powder to create a flavorful lentil soup.

Enjoy this nutrient-packed, flavor-rich dish as a stand-alone meal or as part of a cozy dinner spread. It's comfort food, redefined.

GREEN CHIMICHURRI SAUCE

This quercetin-rich, immunity-boosting sauce is the perfect complement to savory dishes like eggs, roasted vegetables, or grilled proteins. Packed with cilantro—a powerful chelating agent that supports the liver's natural detoxification processes—it's as nutritious as it is flavorful. This vibrant sauce is not only delicious but also loaded with health benefits, making it a versatile addition to any protein dish. Store in an airtight container in the refrigerator for up to 5 days.

1 bunch fresh parsley

1 bunch fresh cilantro

2–3 tablespoons apple cider vinegar

2–3 tablespoons extra virgin olive oil

1 clove garlic

1 tablespoon finely chopped fresh oregano

1 shallot, finely chopped

1. Combine all the ingredients in a food processor or blender.
2. Pulse until the mixture is smooth and well combined. Adjust consistency with a small amount of vinegar or olive oil if needed.
3. Taste and adjust seasoning to your preference.

ADZUKI BEAN AND BROWN RICE BOWL WITH SESAME MISO DRESSING

This bowl is a gut-health powerhouse, packed with fiber, plant-based protein, and fermented ingredients to nourish your microbiome. Adzuki beans are rich in prebiotics, promoting the growth of beneficial gut bacteria, while brown rice provides resistant starch to support digestion. The miso-based dressing offers probiotics to enhance gut diversity, and the addition of fresh, crunchy vegetables delivers antioxidants and digestive enzymes for optimal gut function.

PREP TIME: 15 min
COOK TIME: 30 min (if beans and rice aren't precooked)
SERVES: 2–3

1½ cups cooked adzuki beans
1 cup cooked brown rice
½ large Napa cabbage head, sliced
3 small carrots, shaved
1 cup sugar snap peas, sliced
2 tablespoons sesame seeds
2 tablespoons fresh cilantro, chopped
2 avocados, sliced
1 small fresh red chili, sliced

Sesame Miso Dressing:

¼ cup white miso
⅓ cup rice vinegar
¼ cup olive oil
3 tablespoons tamari
1 tablespoon toasted sesame oil

Mix the adzuki beans and brown rice, layering with fresh Napa cabbage, carrots, and snap peas to create a nutrient-dense base. Top with sesame seeds, cilantro, and avocado slices for added gut support. Combine all the dressing ingredients and drizzle on the beans, blending probiotics and prebiotics to create the ultimate gut-nourishing meal.

How to Make a Really Good Dense Bean Salad

A dense bean salad is incredibly versatile, offering endless ways to combine beans, vegetables, and flavorful dressings. Whether you prefer classic combinations or want to try something new, these recipes highlight how creative and delicious bean salads can be.

CLASSIC DENSE BEAN SALAD

PREP TIME: 15 minutes
COOK TIME: None
SERVES: 4–6

Base Recipe:

1 can (15 oz.) chickpeas, drained and rinsed

1 can (15 oz.) black beans, drained and rinsed

1 can (15 oz.) kidney beans, drained and rinsed

½ cup diced red onion

1 cup chopped bell peppers (any color)

1 cup diced cucumber

1 cup halved cherry tomatoes

¼ cup chopped fresh parsley

2 tablespoons chopped fresh basil

Dressing:

¼ cup olive oil

2 tablespoons lemon juice or apple cider vinegar

1 teaspoon Dijon mustard

1 clove garlic, minced

Salt and pepper to taste

This base recipe is a perfect starting point. Toss everything together and let it marinate for maximum flavor. Optional additions include feta cheese, sesame seeds, or hemp seeds.

Creative Variations for Inspiration

Sun-Dried Tomato Bean Salad

- Add sun-dried tomatoes, artichoke hearts, mozzarella balls, and fresh basil.
- Use white beans and chickpeas as the base.
- This version yields about 5 servings and keeps well in the fridge for up to 4 days.

Buffalo Chicken Bean Salad

- Combine chickpeas, shredded carrots, chopped celery, and grilled chicken.
- Toss with buffalo sauce or a ranch-style dressing for a bold, spicy twist.
- It's like your favorite game-day snack transformed into a nutrient-dense meal.

Late-Summer Bean Salad

- Mix white beans, grilled corn, avocado, cherry tomatoes, and grilled chicken.
- This version is perfect for capturing the fresh flavors of late summer but works year-round.

Green Goddess Bean Salad

- Toss white beans and chickpeas with crunchy vegetables like cucumbers and radishes.
- Drizzle with a blended herb dressing made with parsley, basil, chives, and lemon juice for a fresh, vibrant flavor.
- It's light enough for breakfast and versatile enough to pair with other dishes.

Tips for Making the Best Dense Bean Salad

Choose your beans.

Use a mix of your favorite beans, like chickpeas, black beans, kidney beans, or white beans, for varied texture and flavor.

Add a crunch factor.

Include crunchy veggies like bell peppers, celery, or radishes to balance the creaminess of the beans.

Experiment with dressings.

Go beyond olive oil and vinegar—try herb-based dressings, spicy buffalo sauces, or creamy tahini blends.

Make it a meal.

Add protein like grilled chicken, shrimp, **mozzarella balls,** or for a vegan option, **grilled tofu** to turn your salad into a hearty, satisfying main course.

Dense bean salads are nutrient rich, satisfying, and endlessly customizable. Whether you stick with a classic recipe or explore creative variations, they're an easy way to pack flavor, protein, and fiber into every bite!

A FOODIE'S LUNCH: HOW TO MASTER ANY SALAD

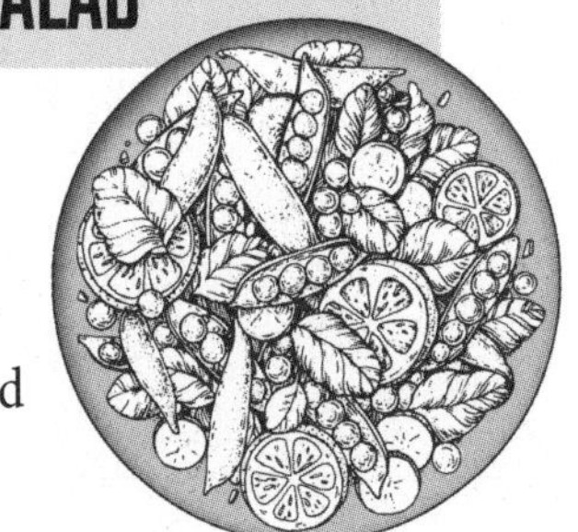

Creating the perfect salad is about balancing flavors, textures, and nutrients. Follow these steps for a #FoodieDietApproved formula to build a versatile, delicious, and nutrient-packed salad tailored to your preferences:

1. Choose a Base

Start with a foundation of fresh, chopped greens to bring flavor, fiber, and micronutrients.

- **Leafy options:** Kale, spinach, butter lettuce, arugula, watercress, mixed greens, iceberg lettuce
- **Crunchy additions:** Cabbage, Brussels sprouts, parsley, dill, cilantro, scallions

2. Add High-Fiber and Polyphenol-Rich Vegetables

Incorporate a mix of raw or cooked veggies to enhance texture, flavor, and antioxidants.

- **Vegetable options:** Beets, carrots, sweet onions, tomatoes, cucumbers, bell peppers, radishes, shallots, celery, artichokes, broccoli, mushrooms, sprouts

3. Include a Protein Source

Boost satiety and make your salad a complete meal with high-quality protein.

- **Animal-based proteins:** Salmon, trout, octopus, shrimp, tuna, sardines, mackerel, eggs, turkey, steak, or chicken

- **Plant-based proteins:** Adzuki beans, chickpeas, lentils, black beans—all types of beans

4. Optional Starchy Grains or Vegetables

Add complex carbs for energy and satisfying texture.

- **Options:** Sweet potatoes, quinoa, rice, buckwheat, purple potatoes

5. Sweet Toppings for Balance

Introduce natural sweetness to complement savory flavors.

- **Fruit options:** Shredded apples, kiwi, pomegranate seeds, blueberries, raspberries, gooseberries

6. Dry and Crunchy Toppings

Add a satisfying crunch with nutrient-dense seeds, nuts, and berries.

- **Options:** Hemp, sunflower, or pumpkin seeds; goji berries, golden berries; walnuts, slivered almonds, pine nuts, sesame seeds

THE SECRET TO A DELICIOUS SALAD IS THE DRESSING

A great dressing can transform any salad, and making it in a mason jar is not only convenient but also ensures everything is perfectly blended with a quick shake. Here's my formula for creating amazing dressings that will wow the crowd, along with some chef-inspired ingredients for extra flair:

1. Start with an oil base

My go-to is extra virgin, wild, cold-pressed olive oil for its rich flavor and health benefits. Other great options include avocado oil for creaminess or sesame oil for a nutty twist.

2. Choose an acid

Add brightness with lemon juice, rice vinegar, apple cider vinegar, or even champagne vinegar for a subtle, refined touch.

3. Pick a thickener

Create a creamy texture with tahini, peanut butter, almond butter, or tamari. For a lighter option, yogurt or buttermilk works wonderfully.

4. Add a sweetener

Balance flavors with a touch of honey, maple syrup, agave syrup, or unsweetened applesauce. Chefs often use pomegranate molasses or fig jam for a unique depth of flavor.

5. Enhance the flavor

Boost complexity with mustard, tamari, fresh herbs like dill or basil, or grated garlic or ginger. Chefs often incorporate anchovy paste for umami or truffle oil for a luxurious finish.

Unique additions for restaurant-worthy dressings:

- **Citrus zest:** Add lemon, lime, or orange zest for a vibrant kick.
- **Fermented ingredients:** Use miso paste or pickled vegetable brine for a tangy, gut-healthy boost.
- **Spices:** Experiment with smoked paprika, sumac, za'atar, or even chili flakes for heat.
- **Cheese:** A bit of grated Parmesan or crumbled blue cheese can add richness and depth.

Shake everything together in the mason jar, and you've got a dressing that will elevate any salad to restaurant-quality perfection!

THE WOW DRESSING

This vibrant dressing combines cilantro's sweet, pungent, and cooling properties to improve digestion, chelate heavy metals, and alkalize the body. Cilantro is also known for its blood-thinning benefits, making this a powerful addition to your meals.

1 bunch fresh cilantro, chopped (including stems)

½ cup raw cashews, soaked overnight

1 tablespoon fresh ginger, minced

2 tablespoons lime juice

2 tablespoons raw honey

¼ teaspoon Himalayan salt

¼ cup water (add more as needed for blending)

Optional: 1–2 tablespoons yogurt and 1 garlic clove for added creaminess and flavor

1. Prepare the dressing. In a small bowl, whisk together the olive oil, apple cider vinegar, Dijon mustard, and honey or maple syrup until emulsified. Season with salt and freshly ground black pepper to taste.
2. Assemble the salad. In a large bowl, combine the sliced radicchio, apple, chopped dates, roasted chickpeas, and chopped parsley. Drizzle the dressing over the salad ingredients and toss gently to combine, ensuring all components are well coated.
3. Serve. Transfer the salad to serving plates and top with shaved Parmesan cheese, if using. Serve immediately.

Serving Suggestions: Drizzle this dressing over salads, roasted vegetables, or grain bowls for a nutrient-packed flavor boost. It also works beautifully as a dip or spread!

GUT-FRIENDLY RADICCHIO SALAD WITH DATES, APPLES, AND ROASTED CHICKPEAS

This gut-friendly salad is a harmonious blend of flavors and textures, featuring radicchio, a bitter leafy green that stimulates digestion and provides antioxidants; apples, rich in fiber and prebiotic pectin to nourish gut bacteria; dates, which add natural sweetness along with fiber and essential minerals; and roasted chickpeas, packed with plant-based protein and fiber to promote satiety and digestive health. A delicious and nutritious addition to your meal repertoire, this recipe is crafted with both taste and wellness in mind.

PREP TIME: 10 minutes
COOK TIME: 15 minutes
SERVES: 2–3

For the salad:

1 head radicchio, cored and thinly sliced

1 apple (such as Honeycrisp or Granny Smith), cored and thinly sliced

½ cup pitted dates, chopped

1 cup roasted chickpeas (store-bought or homemade)

¼ cup shaved Parmesan cheese (optional)

¼ cup chopped fresh parsley

For the dressing:

3 tablespoons extra virgin olive oil

1 tablespoon apple cider vinegar

1 teaspoon Dijon mustard

1 teaspoon honey or maple syrup

Salt and freshly ground black pepper to taste

1. Prepare the dressing. In a small bowl, whisk together the olive oil, apple cider vinegar, Dijon mustard, and honey or maple syrup until emulsified. Season with salt and freshly ground black pepper to taste.
2. Assemble the salad. In a large bowl, combine the sliced radicchio, apple, chopped dates, roasted chickpeas, and chopped parsley. Drizzle the dressing over the salad ingredients and toss gently to combine, ensuring all components are well coated.
3. Serve. Transfer the salad to serving plates and top with shaved Parmesan cheese, if using. Serve immediately.

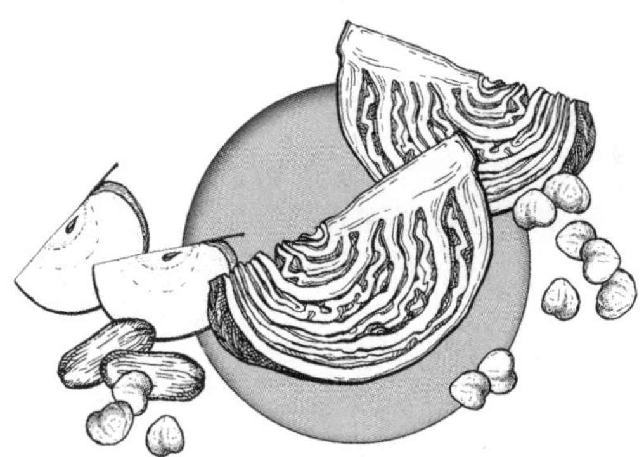

WAIST-SLIMMING RED CABBAGE SALAD

This nutrient-dense red cabbage salad is a motherlode of vitamins, minerals, and antioxidants, designed to support overall health while being light and satisfying. Red cabbage, rich in vitamin C and anthocyanins, promotes healthy digestion and combats inflammation. Beets and carrots add natural sweetness along with beta-carotene and fiber, while cranberries, blueberries, and kiwi or apple provide a burst of antioxidants and gut-friendly benefits. Topped with omega-3-rich walnuts and hemp seeds, this salad offers a balanced blend of flavor, crunch, and nutrition.

PREP TIME: 15 minutes
COOKING TIME: 20 minutes
SERVES: 4

1 medium red cabbage (outer leaves removed, trimmed, and coarsely chopped)

1 small beet (peeled and shredded)

2 medium carrots (peeled and shredded)

½ small red onion (thinly sliced)

1 kiwi or 1 apple (sliced)

¼ cup dried cranberries

1 tablespoon capers

¼ cup walnuts (chopped)

1 tablespoon hemp seeds

½ cup apple cider vinegar

¼ teaspoon salt

¼ cup olive oil

¼ cup fresh blueberries

1. In a large bowl, combine the red cabbage, shredded beet, shredded carrots, sliced onion, kiwi or apple, cranberries, capers, walnuts, hemp seeds, and blueberries.
2. In a small bowl, whisk together the apple cider vinegar, olive oil, and salt to create the dressing.
3. Pour the dressing over the salad mixture. Toss well to coat all the ingredients evenly.
4. Cover the bowl and refrigerate for at least an hour or overnight to allow the flavors to meld.

PRO TIP: Letting the salad marinate enhances the flavor and softens the cabbage, making it even more delicious and easy to digest.

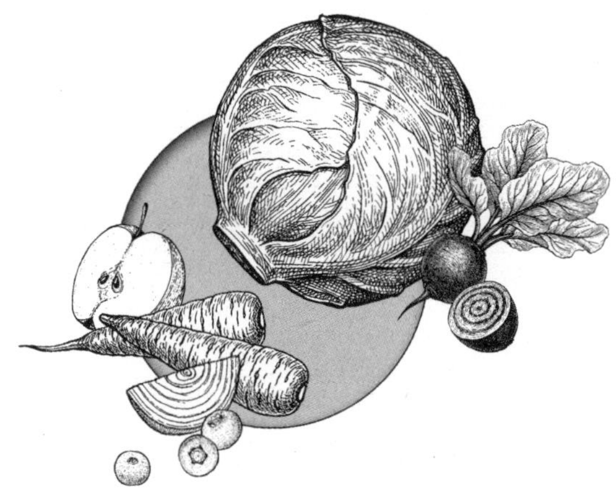

TURMERIC-INFUSED QUINOA SALAD

This vibrant quinoa salad combines nutrient-rich ingredients with bold flavors for a dish that's both satisfying and nourishing. The quinoa, cooked in bone broth with turmeric, provides a flavorful and anti-inflammatory base, while fresh vegetables, beans, and herbs elevate this salad into a nutrient extravaganza.

PREP TIME: 15 minutes
COOK TIME: 15 minutes
SERVES: 4

1 cup quinoa, cooked in 2 cups bone broth with 1 teaspoon turmeric

2 cups fresh kale, chopped (stems removed)

1 bell pepper, diced (any color)

1 avocado, diced

1 cup cherry tomatoes, halved

1 cup beans (black beans, chickpeas, or your choice)

2 tablespoons sesame seeds

2 scallions, thinly sliced

¼ cup fresh cilantro, chopped

¼ cup olives (Kalamata or green), halved

Dressing:

2 tablespoons fresh lemon juice

2 tablespoons extra virgin olive oil

1 clove garlic, minced

1 tablespoon apple cider vinegar

Salt and black pepper to taste

1. Cook the quinoa. Rinse the quinoa thoroughly, then cook it in bone broth with turmeric according to package instructions. Once cooked, fluff with a fork and let it cool.
2. Prepare the vegetables.
3. In a large bowl, massage the chopped kale with a small drizzle of olive oil and a pinch of salt until slightly softened.
4. Add the diced bell pepper, avocado, cherry tomatoes, beans, sesame seeds, scallions, cilantro, and olives.
5. Make the dressing. In a small bowl, whisk together the lemon juice, olive oil, minced garlic, apple cider vinegar, salt, and pepper.
6. Assemble the salad.
7. Add the cooled quinoa to the bowl with the vegetables.
8. Pour the dressing over the salad and toss gently to combine.
9. Serve. Transfer the salad to a serving dish and sprinkle with additional sesame seeds or fresh herbs, if desired.

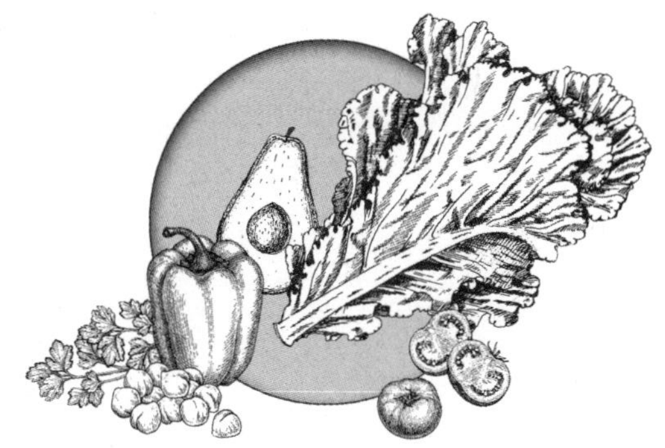

Gut-Healing Recipes

In this section, you'll find a curated collection of nourishing recipes designed to support digestion, reduce inflammation, and restore gut integrity. Each dish features gut-friendly ingredients—like fermented foods, healing herbs, fiber-rich vegetables, and balanced proteins—to help you optimize microbiome health and feel your best from the inside out. Whether you're managing symptoms or simply eating for prevention, these meals are both functional and flavorful.

ITALIAN VEGGIE DIP WITH ANCHOVIES

This Italian-inspired veggie dip is bursting with bold flavors and powerful nutrients. Packed with omega-3-rich anchovies, anti-inflammatory herbs, and medicinal garlic, it's a heart-healthy and immune-boosting addition to your snack or appetizer lineup. Best of all, it's simple to make and pairs perfectly with gluten-free crackers or fresh vegetable crudités.

PREP TIME: 10 minutes
COOK TIME: None
SERVES: 4

1 bunch parsley

½ can anchovies

2 cloves garlic

1 teaspoon capers

2 tablespoons olive oil

2 tablespoons apple cider vinegar

1 tablespoon mustard

Pepper to taste

1. Combine ingredients. Place all ingredients in a food processor.
2. Blend until smooth. Pulse until the mixture becomes a creamy, smooth dip.
3. Serve. Transfer the dip to a bowl and serve with gluten-free crackers or a colorful assortment of vegetable crudités like carrots, celery, and bell peppers.

SIMPLE BONE BROTH–BASED BROCCOLI SOUP

This nourishing broccoli soup is made with bone broth, creating a rich, gut-healing base. Packed with vitamins, minerals, and collagen, it's a simple and comforting recipe that supports digestion and detoxification and is a perfect option for a light meal or an appetizer, delivering warmth and nutrients with every spoonful.

PREP TIME: 10 minutes
COOK TIME: 20 minutes
SERVES: 2–3

1 tablespoon olive oil or ghee

1 small onion, diced

2 garlic cloves, minced

4 cups broccoli florets (about 1 large head)

3 cups bone broth (chicken or beef)

1 cup unsweetened coconut milk or heavy cream (optional, for creaminess)

Salt and black pepper to taste

1 tablespoon fresh lemon juice (optional, for brightness)

Fresh parsley or chives, chopped (for garnish)

1. Sauté aromatics. Heat olive oil in a large pot over medium heat. Add the onion and garlic, and sauté until softened and fragrant, for 3 to 4 minutes.
2. Add broccoli and bone broth. Add the broccoli florets to the pot and pour in the bone broth. Bring to a gentle boil, then reduce the heat and simmer for 10 to 12 minutes, or until the broccoli is tender.
3. Blend the soup. Use an immersion blender to purée the soup until smooth, or, once cooled, transfer the mixture to a blender in batches.
4. Adjust consistency. If desired, stir in coconut milk for a creamy texture. Season with salt and black pepper to taste.
5. Finish and serve. Stir in the lemon juice (if using) and ladle the soup into bowls. Garnish with fresh parsley or chives.

SAUTÉED LEEKS WITH GHEE AND GOAT CHEESE

Deliciously simple gut-healing leeks are a prebiotic-rich vegetable that nourishes beneficial gut bacteria and a healthy microbiome. Ghee, with its high concentration of butyrate, supports gut lining repair and reduces inflammation while goat cheese provides probiotics to further enhance microbiome diversity. Together, these ingredients work synergistically to heal and strengthen the gut lining while delivering an appetizer that's both comforting and sophisticated.

PREP TIME: 10 minutes
COOK TIME: 10 minutes
SERVES: 4

3 large leeks, trimmed and cleaned (white and light green parts only)

2 tablespoons ghee

½ teaspoon sea salt

Freshly ground black pepper to taste

2 ounces goat cheese, crumbled

1 tablespoon fresh thyme leaves (optional, for garnish)

1 teaspoon lemon zest (optional, for brightness)

1. Prepare the leeks. Slice the leeks lengthwise and then into 2-inch segments. Rinse thoroughly to remove any grit or dirt.
2. Sauté the leeks:
3. Heat the ghee in a large skillet over medium heat. Once melted and hot, add the leeks in a single layer.
4. Sprinkle with salt and a few grinds of black pepper.
5. Cook for 5 to 7 minutes, stirring occasionally, until the leeks are softened and starting to caramelize.
6. Transfer the sautéed leeks to a serving plate while still warm.
7. Scatter the crumbled goat cheese over the top, allowing it to soften slightly from the heat of the leeks.
8. Optional garnish. Sprinkle with fresh thyme leaves and a touch of lemon zest for added flavor and visual appeal.
9. Serve immediately as a warm appetizer with crusty gluten-free bread or alongside vegetable crudités for dipping.

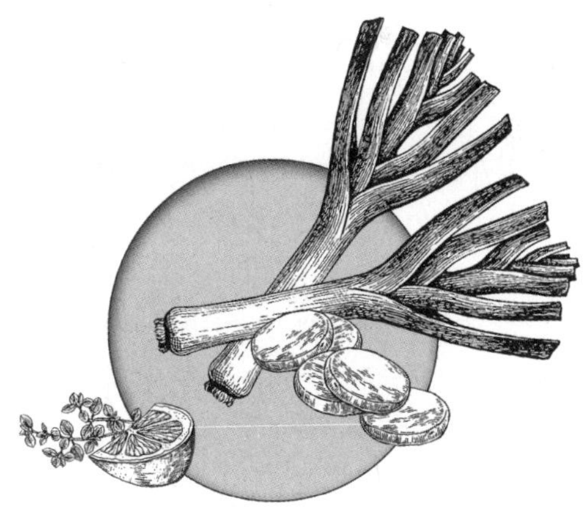

HOMEMADE TURMERIC SAUERKRAUT

Pair this turmeric-infused sauerkraut with your eggs or avocado toast to add a flavorful boost to your meals while delivering probiotics with anti-inflammatory benefits. Enjoy it as a side dish, in sandwiches, or atop salads for added zest and probiotics.

PREP TIME: 20 minutes
FERMENTATION TIME: 7–21 days
SERVES: 16 servings (1–2 tablespoons per serving)

1 small head of cabbage

2–3 teaspoons of sea salt

2½ teaspoons dried turmeric or freshly grated turmeric

½ teaspoon ground black pepper

1 large clove of garlic, grated

1–2 inches of fresh ginger root, grated

½ jalapeño pepper, finely chopped or grated (optional)

1. Prepare the cabbage. Remove and set aside a large outer leaf from the cabbage. Finely shred the remaining cabbage using a mandolin slicer or grater.
2. Combine ingredients. In a large bowl, mix the shredded cabbage with salt, turmeric, black pepper, garlic, ginger, and jalapeño (if using). Massage the mixture thoroughly to release the cabbage's natural juices, creating a brine.
3. Pack the jar. Firmly pack the cabbage mixture into a clean glass jar, ensuring it's submerged under its own brine to promote anaerobic fermentation. Place the reserved cabbage leaf on top to keep the shredded cabbage submerged.
4. Fermentation. Seal the jar with a lid and store it at room temperature, away from direct sunlight. Allow the sauerkraut to ferment for at least 7 days. Taste periodically until it reaches your desired level of tanginess.
5. Storage. Once fermented to your liking, refrigerate the sauerkraut to slow fermentation. It can be stored in the refrigerator for several months.

GOLDEN CAULIFLOWER BUDDHA BOWL

This bowl provides complete protein while supporting detoxification. The fat in tahini helps absorb turmeric's benefits.

PREP TIME: 10 minutes
COOK TIME: 25 minutes
SERVES: 2

For the bowl:

1 head cauliflower, cut into florets

1 can chickpeas, drained

2 tablespoons avocado oil

1 cup cooked quinoa

2 cups baby spinach

For the spice mix:

2 teaspoons turmeric

1 teaspoon cumin

½ teaspoon coriander

Black pepper

For the dressing:

¼ cup tahini

1 lemon, juiced

1 garlic clove, minced

Hot water to thin, if needed

1. Toss cauliflower and chickpeas with oil and spice mix.
2. Roast at 425°F for 25 minutes, stirring halfway.
3. Whisk tahini dressing ingredients until smooth.
4. Layer bowls: quinoa, spinach, roasted vegetables.
5. Drizzle with dressing.

SURPRISINGLY DELICIOUS BROCCOLI SALAD

This broccoli salad not only is delicious but also offers a versatile way to use up lingering vegetables in your fridge. You can substitute or add celery, Brussels sprouts, carrots, radishes, spinach, or arugula for a personalized twist. Packed with crunchy textures and a tangy tamari dressing, this salad is perfect as a side dish or light meal.

PREP TIME: 10 minutes
COOK TIME: None
SERVES: 4

For the salad:

1 small head broccoli

1 cup green beans, trimmed

1 cup red or green cabbage, thinly sliced

1 cup cooked, shredded chicken (optional, for added protein)

For the dressing:

2 tablespoons tamari (or soy sauce)

1 tablespoon rice vinegar

2 tablespoons olive oil

1 teaspoon honey or pure maple syrup

1. Prepare vegetables. Bring a pot of water to a boil. Cut small florets from the broccoli stalk. Use a vegetable peeler to remove the tough outer peel from the stalk, then thinly slice it. Into the boiling water, put the broccoli florets, stalk, and green beans, blanching them for about 1 minute until bright green. Immediately transfer the vegetables to an ice bath to stop the cooking process. Once cooled, drain and blot dry with a clean towel.
2. Assemble the salad. In a large bowl, combine the sliced cabbage, blanched broccoli, green beans, and shredded chicken (if using).
3. Make the dressing. In a small bowl, whisk together the tamari, rice vinegar, olive oil, and honey until well combined.
4. Dress and toss. Pour the dressing over the salad ingredients and toss until evenly coated.
5. Serve. Let the salad sit for 5 to 10 minutes to allow the flavors to meld, then serve immediately.

Optional additions:

- Toasted sesame seeds or sliced almonds for crunch
- Chopped fresh herbs like cilantro or parsley for extra flavor
- A sprinkle of red pepper flakes for a hint of spice

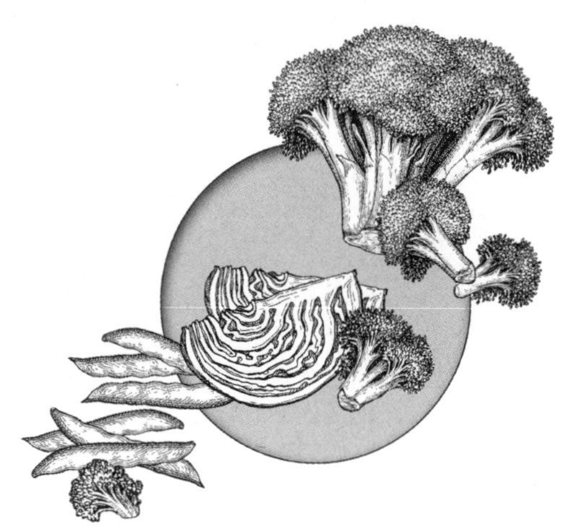

HEALTHIEST BORSCHT RECIPE

The New York University Food Lab features this delicious borscht recipe, and I made it for a cooking segment on a news channel because it is simple and nutritious. It makes for a heartwarming and comforting meal that's even better the next day! The secret lies in simmering the vegetables, allowing their flavors to meld into a rich, nourishing soup. This traditional Russian winter soup is both delicious and packed with fiber from the vegetables, along with collagen and amino acids from the bone broth. Whether enjoyed fresh or the next day, this borscht is sure to warm your heart and nourish your body. *Bon appétit!*

PREP TIME: 15 minutes
COOK TIME: 25 minutes
SERVES: 5–6

2 medium beets, peeled and cut into cubes

2 medium potatoes, peeled and cut into cubes

2 carrots, peeled and cut into cubes

1 tablespoon olive oil or avocado oil

1 onion, chopped

2 garlic cloves, minced

1 quart bone broth (@Bonafide or any high-quality brand)

1 cup shredded cabbage

Salt and pepper to taste

Sour cream or plain yogurt (for serving)

1 teaspoon of fresh herbs (dill recommended) as garnish

1. Prep the vegetables. Peel and chop the beets, potatoes, and carrots into bite-size cubes.
2. Sauté aromatics. In a large skillet, heat olive oil over medium heat. Sauté the onion and garlic until fragrant and translucent.
3. Cook the vegetables. Add the chopped beets, potatoes, and carrots to the skillet with the sautéed onion and garlic. Cook for 10 minutes, stirring occasionally.
4. Simmer the soup. Transfer the vegetable mixture to a large pot and pour in the bone broth. Add the shredded cabbage.
5. Simmer everything together over medium heat for 15 to 20 minutes, or until the vegetables are tender.
6. Add salt and pepper to taste. Ladle the borscht into bowls and swirl in a dollop of sour cream or plain yogurt. Garnish with fresh dill.

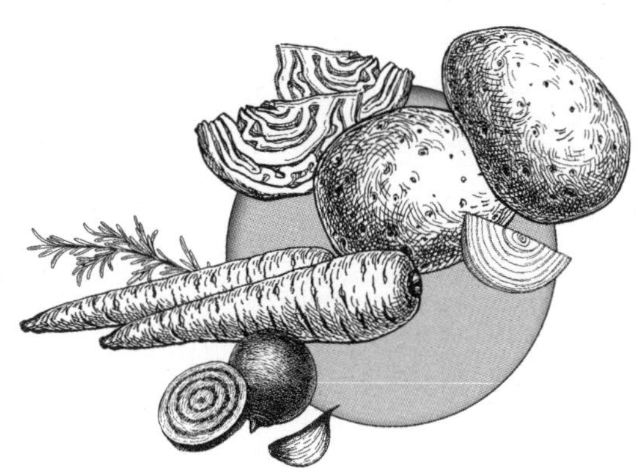

EASY CARROT GINGER SOUP

Packed with nutrient-rich carrots, immune-boosting ginger, and anti-inflammatory turmeric, this warming soup is low in fat and full of healing benefits. It's perfect for a healthy lunch or dinner, supporting digestion and overall immunity with every sip.

PREP TIME: 10 minutes
COOK TIME: 25 minutes
SERVES: 3

2 tablespoons extra virgin olive oil

½ cup white onion, diced

2 cloves garlic, minced

3 large carrots, peeled and cubed

1 cup celeriac root, peeled and cubed

Himalayan salt, a pinch

4 cups low-sodium vegetable broth

1 inch fresh ginger root, peeled and sliced

1 teaspoon turmeric powder

1 teaspoon ground cumin

Cayenne pepper, a pinch

Cumin or fresh parsley for garnish

1. Sauté the aromatics. Heat olive oil in a large saucepan over medium heat. Add diced onion and minced garlic. Cook for 3 to 4 minutes, stirring often, until the onion is translucent but not browned.
2. Cook the vegetables. Add carrots and celeriac root to the pot. Sprinkle with a pinch of salt and cook, stirring frequently, for 1 minute to soften slightly without browning.
3. Simmer the soup. Pour in the vegetable broth and bring to a boil. Add the ginger, lower heat to a simmer, cover, and cook for 20 minutes, or until the carrots and celeriac are tender.
4. Blend the soup. Remove from heat and let cool slightly. Purée the soup in a blender until smooth, then return it to the pot.
5. Season. Stir in the turmeric, cumin, and cayenne pepper. Taste and adjust seasoning with more salt if needed.
6. Pour the soup into bowls and garnish with a sprinkle of cumin and/or fresh parsley.

BELLISSIMO ITALIAN VEGETABLE SOUP

This hearty and flavorful vegetable soup is packed with nutrient-dense ingredients and a delicious balance of spices. It's perfect for a comforting meal while providing anti-inflammatory and immune-boosting benefits.

PREP TIME: 10 minutes
COOK TIME: 25 minutes
SERVES: 4

3 tablespoons olive oil

2 cloves garlic, minced

1 medium white onion, chopped

3 stalks celery, chopped

2 carrots, chopped

2 stalks leeks, sliced

1-inch piece raw turmeric, grated

3 leaves fresh sage

1 sweet potato, diced

1 cup broccoli florets

1 cup cauliflower florets

2 cups bone broth

1 handful spinach

1 bunch parsley, chopped

1. Sauté aromatics:
   - Heat olive oil in a deep cast-iron pan over medium heat.
   - Add garlic, onion, celery, carrots, and leeks. Sauté until softened and fragrant, for about 5 minutes.
2. Stir in turmeric and sage. Cook for another 3 minutes to release the flavors.
3. Simmer vegetables. Add sweet potatoes, broccoli, cauliflower, and bone broth. Bring to a gentle simmer and cook for 10 to 15 minutes, or until the vegetables are tender.
4. Finish with greens. During the last 5 minutes, add spinach and parsley. Stir well to combine.
5. Blend to desired consistency:
6. Remove the soup from heat and let it cool slightly for about 20 minutes.
7. Using an immersion blender, blend the soup until it reaches your desired consistency—smooth or slightly chunky.
8. Serve. Ladle into bowls and enjoy warm. Pair with a slice of crusty bread or enjoy as is for a wholesome meal.

SIMPLE AND OH-SO-DELICIOUS LENTIL SOUP

This hearty lentil soup is packed with flavor, nutrition, and vibrant greens, making it an excellent comfort meal. Lentils are rich in plant-based protein, fiber, and essential minerals while turmeric, spinach, and herbs provide anti-inflammatory and antioxidant benefits.

PREP TIME: 10 minutes
COOK TIME: 25 minutes
SERVES: 4

2 tablespoons extra virgin olive oil

1 large onion, diced

2 stalks celery, diced

1 large carrot, diced

½ teaspoon dried thyme

½ teaspoon dried oregano

¼ teaspoon turmeric

3 cloves garlic, minced

1 cup lentils (green, red, or split mung)

1 teaspoon sea salt

½ teaspoon black pepper

½ pound spinach

½ bunch cilantro or parsley, coarsely chopped, for garnish

Optional: turkey bacon, cooked and crumbled

1. Sauté the aromatics. Heat olive oil in a medium-size soup pot over medium heat. Add the onion and sauté until translucent, for about 3 to 5 minutes. Add the celery and carrot, cooking for another 3 to 5 minutes.
2. Add spices and lentils. Stir in thyme, oregano, turmeric, and garlic. Add the lentils and 5 cups of water.
3. Simmer the soup. Bring the mixture to a boil, then lower heat to a simmer. Cover and cook for 20 to 30 minutes, or until the lentils are creamy and tender.
4. Adjust consistency. Add more water if needed to reach your desired consistency.
5. Finish with greens. Stir in salt, pepper, and spinach. Cook for another 2 to 3 minutes, or until the spinach is wilted. Adjust seasoning to taste.
6. Serve. Garnish with chopped cilantro and turkey bacon (if using) for extra flavor. Serve warm and enjoy!

ROASTED BEET AND WALNUT SALAD

This vibrant salad combines the earthy sweetness of roasted beets, the tangy creaminess of probiotic yogurt, the natural sweetness of prunes, and the satisfying crunch of walnuts. Packed with fiber, antioxidants, and probiotics, it's a simple yet powerful dish to support gut health and overall wellness. Beets aid detoxification, walnuts provide healthy fats, and yogurt contributes beneficial bacteria to nourish your microbiome. Great as a side dish or a light meal, this recipe is as delicious as it is nutritious!

PREP TIME: 10 minutes
COOK TIME: 20 minutes
SERVES: 4

2–3 medium-size beets

5–7 prunes

Handful of walnuts

½ cup plain probiotic yogurt

1. Roast the beets. Preheat your oven to 450°F (232°C). Wrap the beets in parchment paper and roast for 40 minutes, or until tender.
2. Prep the beets. Once cooled, peel the beets and finely chop or shred them.
3. Prepare the prunes. Soak the prunes in hot water until softened. Remove the pits and chop them into small pieces.
4. Add walnuts. Chop the walnuts into smaller pieces.
5. Combine ingredients. In a bowl, mix the roasted beets, chopped prunes, and walnuts. Top with plain probiotic yogurt for a creamy, tangy finish.
6. Serve. Enjoy immediately or let chill for 15 to 20 minutes to allow the flavors to meld.

Hormone-Balancing Breakfast Ideas

HERB-LOADED FRITTATA

Choline-rich eggs combined with herbs provide brain-boosting nutrients. Perfect for breakfast-for-dinner or using leftover vegetables.

PREP TIME: 10 minutes
COOK TIME: 15 minutes
SERVES: 4

8 pasture-raised eggs

¼ cup full-fat coconut milk or cream

1 cup mixed fresh herbs (parsley, dill, chives, basil)

Sea salt and pepper to taste

2 tablespoons ghee

2 cups leftover roasted vegetables

¼ cup goat cheese (optional)

1. Whisk eggs with coconut milk, most herbs (save some for garnish), salt, and pepper.
2. Heat ghee in oven-safe skillet over medium heat.
3. Add vegetables, warm through.
4. Pour egg mixture over the vegetables, cook until edges set (for 3 to 4 minutes).
5. Top with goat cheese, if using, and broil for 3 to 5 minutes, until golden.

HOMEMADE SALMON LOX RECIPE

Homemade lox with wild-caught salmon is perfect for breakfast eggs, salads, or as a gourmet appetizer.

PREP TIME: 10 minutes
COOK TIME: 2 days
SERVES: 4

3–4 ounces wild Alaskan salmon (defrosted if frozen)

Fresh or dried dill, finely chopped

3 teaspoons sea salt

Optional: Smoked or truffle salt, black pepper, fresh lemon slices

1. Prepare the salmon. Defrost the salmon if frozen and pat it dry. Finely chop the fresh dill.
2. Season the salmon. In a glass storage container, rub the salmon generously with a mixture of sea salt, dill, and optional ingredients like black pepper or smoked salt. If desired, add lemon slices for an extra zesty flavor.
3. Wrap and cure. Lay a large piece of plastic wrap on a flat surface. Place the salmon skin-side down on the wrap. Wrap the salmon tightly, ensuring it is fully enclosed, and place it in a container with a lid. Cover the container and refrigerate for 2 days.
4. Rinse and slice. After 2 days, remove the salmon from the fridge and rinse it under cold water to remove excess salt. Pat dry and thinly slice the salmon.
5. Serve or store. Serve the salmon immediately, or transfer it to a clean container, cover, and refrigerate until ready to serve.

BONUS TIP: Save the skin. Don't discard the salmon skin! Fry it into crispy salmon bacon for a delicious and nutritious snack.

GLUTEN-FREE, PROTEIN-PACKED GRAIN-FREE WAFFLES

This recipe is grain-free and packed with protein from almond flour, pea protein, and yogurt, making it an excellent option for weight loss or maintenance while satisfying your sweet cravings. For added flavor, sprinkle in a pinch of cinnamon or nutmeg.

PREP TIME: 10 minutes
COOK TIME: 15 minutes
SERVES: 4

2 tablespoons cassava flour

3 tablespoons almond flour

1 tablespoon pea protein powder

1 teaspoon vanilla extract

1 teaspoon baking powder

1 cup plain yogurt (protein-rich and probiotic-packed)

2 large eggs

1. In a mixing bowl, whisk together all the ingredients until smooth and well combined.
2. Preheat your waffle maker. Lightly grease if necessary.
3. Pour about 3 tablespoons of batter onto the waffle maker for each waffle.
4. Cook until the waffles are golden brown and crispy.
5. Serve warm with honey or maple syrup and fresh berries for a naturally sweet and nutritious topping.

COCONUT CHIA SEED PUDDING WITH COLLAGEN

This creamy, nutrient-packed pudding is a perfect protein-rich option for breakfast or a snack, offering a balance of fiber, omega-3 fatty acids, and healthy fats from chia seeds, one of the most nutrient-dense plant-based foods. Boosted with grass-fed collagen for added protein, this breakfast dish supports muscle repair, healthy skin, and overall vitality while keeping you full and energized throughout the day. Naturally gluten-free and rich in antioxidants, this pudding can be made ahead and customized with fresh fruit and cultured coconut yogurt for a complete, well-rounded meal.

PREP TIME: 5 minutes
COOK TIME: 2–4 minutes
SERVES: 4

1 can (13.5 oz.) organic full-fat coconut milk

1 tablespoon honey or maple syrup (adjust to taste)

½ teaspoon vanilla extract

1–2 scoops collagen powder (unflavored or vanilla)

½ cup chia seeds

Optional Toppings:

Fresh or frozen blueberries and raspberries

Slices of banana

Spoonful of cultured coconut yogurt

1. In a medium bowl, whisk together the coconut milk, honey, vanilla extract, and collagen powder until smooth.
2. Add the chia seeds and stir well to combine, ensuring there are no clumps.
3. Cover the bowl and refrigerate for at least 4 hours or overnight, allowing the pudding to set and thicken.
4. Before serving, give the pudding a good stir. Divide it into bowls or jars and add your favorite toppings, such as fresh berries, banana slices, or a dollop of cultured coconut yogurt.

Superfood Smoothies

ELLA'S EXTRALICIOUS ANTIOXIDANT BERRY SMOOTHIE PARFAIT

Packed with antioxidants and protein, this smoothie parfait offers a real boost to start your day. The combination of plant-based protein, berries, and nutrient-dense seeds supports immunity, energy, and overall health. Enjoy this delicious, nourishing breakfast and share it with your loved ones!

1 cup mixed berries (blueberries and raspberries)

1 medium red apple (or banana)

1 small beet

1-inch piece fresh ginger, peeled

1 tablespoon almond butter

1 scoop pea protein powder (or collagen powder)

1–2 cups plant-based milk (flax, cashew, almond, or hemp)

1 tablespoon hemp, chia, or flax seeds

Optional: 1 date (for added sweetness) and granola (for added crunch)

1. Blend all ingredients in a high-speed blender until smooth.
2. Serve with plain Bulgarian or Greek probiotic yogurt for a gut-healthy protein boost.
3. Optional: Top with granola for added crunch.

COLLAGEN BLUEBERRY SMOOTHIE

1 cup wild blueberries

2 scoops collagen peptides

1 handful spinach

1 tablespoon almond butter

1 cup unsweetened coconut milk

¼ avocado

1 tablespoon chia seeds

1. Combine all ingredients in a high-speed blender.
2. Blend until smooth and creamy.
3. Add more liquid if needed for desired consistency.

PRO TIP: Wild blueberries have two to three times more antioxidants than the conventional fruit. Collagen combined with vitamin C–rich berries maximizes absorption.

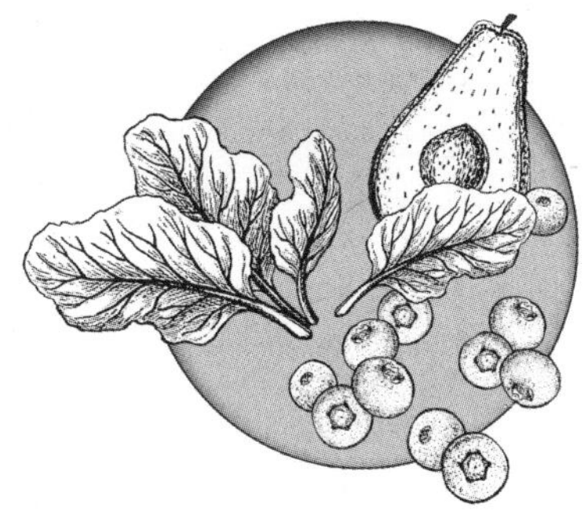

VERY BERRY COLLAGEN SMOOTHIE RECIPE

½ cup fresh or frozen blueberries

½ cup fresh or frozen cranberries

1 tablespoon almond butter

1 scoop grass-fed collagen powder

1 handful fresh spinach

½ banana (for natural creaminess)

1 cup water

Optional: ice cubes

1. Place all ingredients in a blender: blueberries, cranberries, almond butter, collagen powder, spinach, banana, water, and ice (if using).
2. Blend on high until smooth and creamy, for 30–60 seconds.
3. Pour into a glass and enjoy immediately!

PRO TIP: Adding half a banana not only enhances creaminess but also provides a natural touch of sweetness, perfectly balancing the tartness of cranberries.

GREEN GODDESS SMOOTHIE

This Green Goddess Smoothie is crafted to support liver detoxification and promote optimal gut health. The combination of chlorophyll-rich greens, hydrating cucumber, and the digestion-stimulating effects of ginger and lemon work synergistically to enhance bile production, flush out toxins, and strengthen the intestinal lining.

1 handful fresh spinach

1 handful fresh kale or Swiss chard (stems removed)

½ cucumber, chopped

1 small lemon, juiced

1-inch piece fresh ginger, peeled and grated

1 green apple, chopped

1 cup unsweetened coconut water or water

½ avocado

Optional: ice cubes

1. Place spinach, kale, cucumber, lemon juice, ginger, green apple, coconut water, and avocado in a blender.
2. Blend on high speed until smooth and creamy. Add ice cubes if you prefer a chilled smoothie.
3. Taste and adjust the consistency with more water if needed, or add a touch more lemon for extra zing.
4. Pour into a glass and enjoy immediately.

Low-Sugar Desserts

TWO-INGREDIENT IMMUNE-BOOSTING GUMMIES

This immune-boosting gummy recipe was a crowd-pleaser when I made it on TV, and I later learned that Gisele Bündchen uses a similar version for her children. Packed with collagen, gelatin, and elderberry, these gummies are a fun, portable way to support gut, skin, and immune health—plus they're naturally sweetened with pomegranate juice, making them delicious and nutritious at the same time.

PREP TIME: 5 minutes
COOK TIME: 2–3 hours
SERVES: 4

2 cups 100 percent pure pomegranate juice (unsweetened)

2 tablespoons grass-fed gelatin powder

2 tablespoons elderberry syrup

Optional: 1–2 scoops grass-fed collagen powder for extra benefits

1. Bloom the gelatin. In a small bowl, combine ½ cup of pomegranate juice with the gelatin powder. Stir gently and let it sit for 5 minutes to "bloom." This step ensures smooth and evenly textured gummies.
2. Heat and dissolve. Warm the remaining 1½ cups of pomegranate juice in a small saucepan over medium heat (do not boil). Remove from heat and stir in the bloomed gelatin until completely dissolved.
3. Add the elderberry and collagen. Stir in the elderberry syrup and collagen powder (if using) until fully incorporated.
4. Pour into molds. Carefully pour the mixture into silicone gummy molds or a shallow glass dish if molds aren't available.

5. Set and chill. Refrigerate the molds for 2 to 3 hours, or until the gummies are firm and set.
6. Pop and enjoy. Remove gummies from the molds or cut into bite-size pieces if using a dish.

These gummies combine the structural benefits of gelatin and collagen, which support gut integrity, enhance skin elasticity, and promote joint health while also providing a chewy texture that makes them fun to eat. The pomegranate juice delivers a potent dose of antioxidants and polyphenols, offering protective benefits for both immune function and cardiovascular health. Elderberry syrup, renowned for its antiviral properties, adds an immune-boosting edge, particularly valuable during cold and flu season. These nutrient-dense, easy-to-carry gummies are a practical and flavorful way to fortify your body's defenses and maintain vitality throughout the year.

HEALTHY NUTELLA SPREAD WITH COLLAGEN

This recipe is protein-rich, supports stable blood sugar, and promotes healthy skin.

PREP TIME: 10 minutes
COOK TIME: none
MAKES: 1 cup

2 cups hazelnuts, roasted

2 scoops chocolate collagen peptides

2 tablespoons raw cacao powder

2 to 3 tablespoons monk fruit sweetener

¼ teaspoon vanilla extract

Pinch of sea salt

1 to 2 tablespoons coconut oil

1. Process hazelnuts in food processor until smooth and buttery (for 5 to 7 minutes).
2. Add remaining ingredients except coconut oil; process until combined.
3. Stream in coconut oil until desired consistency is reached.
4. Store in airtight container in refrigerator.

PRO TIP: This spread provides sustained energy without blood sugar spikes. Perfect on grain-free bread or with apple slices for a balanced snack.

SIMPLY DELICIOUS STEWED APPLES

Simple and sugar-free, these stewed apples make a delicious topping for yogurt, oatmeal, or pancakes, or can be enjoyed on their own as a satisfying dessert or snack. The almond butter adds a creamy richness and boosts the protein content while the cinnamon and lemon juice enhance the natural sweetness of the apples.

PREP TIME: 7 minutes
COOK TIME: 25 minutes
SERVES: 4

3 apples, cored and sliced or diced

1 tablespoon ghee

1 tablespoon lemon juice

½ teaspoon cinnamon

Yogurt for serving

Toppings:
Almond butter
Honey
Chopped walnuts

1. Prepare the apples. Remove the core from the apples, then slice or dice them to your preferred size.
2. Melt the ghee in a pan over medium heat. Add the apples and sauté for 2 to 3 minutes, stirring occasionally.
3. Pour in the lemon juice and sprinkle with cinnamon. Stir to combine, and let the apples cook for an additional 5 to 7 minutes until tender.
4. Serve. Spoon the warm stewed apples over yogurt. Drizzle with almond butter and honey, then sprinkle with chopped walnuts for added texture and flavor.

BLACK BEAN BROWNIES

A decadent, healthier twist on a classic dessert but with a secret ingredient. Serve them first, then reveal the surprising *black bean base!* Most people won't believe how rich and fudgy they taste. These brownies are naturally gluten-free and packed with fiber and protein from the black beans, making them a guilt-free indulgence.

PREP TIME: 10 minutes
COOK TIME: 18 minutes
SERVES: 9–12 squares

1 can black beans (drained and well-rinsed)

2 tablespoons cocoa powder

½ cup old-fashioned oats

¼ teaspoon salt

⅓ cup pure maple syrup or honey

¼ cup coconut oil or ghee

2 teaspoons pure vanilla extract

½ teaspoon baking powder

½ to ⅔ cup chocolate chips

Optional: Additional chocolate chips for topping

1. Preheat and prepare. Preheat your oven to 350°F (175°C). Lightly grease an 8×8-inch baking pan or line it with parchment paper.
2. Blend the batter. Combine all ingredients except the chocolate chips in a food processor. Blend until completely smooth, ensuring no lumps for the best texture and flavor. *Note:* A blender can be used if necessary, but a food processor yields the best results.
3. Mix and pour. Stir in the chocolate chips, then pour the batter into the prepared pan. Smooth the top with a spatula. If desired, sprinkle extra chocolate chips over the top for a decorative touch.
4. Bake for 15 to 18 minutes, or until the edges are set and the center is slightly firm.
5. Let the brownies cool for at least 10 minutes before cutting. If they appear undercooked, refrigerate them overnight to allow them to firm up.

GOLDEN LATTE

This comforting caffeine- and dairy-free, anti-inflammatory drink is warmed with aromatic turmeric and cinnamon, deliciously supporting digestion and immunity.

1 cup unsweetened plant-based milk (almond, oat, or coconut)

½ teaspoon ground turmeric

⅛ teaspoon ground cinnamon

½ teaspoon raw honey or maple syrup

¼ teaspoon vanilla extract

Pinch of black pepper

Pinch of ginger powder

1. Blend all ingredients in a high-speed blender until smooth and frothy.
2. Pour into a small saucepan, heat over medium heat for 3 to 5 minutes until hot but not boiling.
3. Pour into your favorite mug and enjoy.

PRO TIP: Black pepper increases turmeric absorption by 2,000 percent. Enjoy this before bed to reduce inflammation or as an afternoon pick-me-up.

ELECTROLYTE HYDRATION LEMONADE

There's nothing like homemade lemonade on a hot summer day! This gut-healthy, refreshing, and comforting drink is high in electrolytes and sweetened with honey. Optional mint and blueberries add even more flavor!

1 large lemon, juiced

2 tablespoons raw honey

4 cups water

1 cup ice (optional)

1 tablespoon apple cider vinegar

1 sprig mint leaves, chopped (optional)

1 tablespoon frozen wild organic blueberries (optional)

1 pinch Celtic sea salt

1. Blend the berry mixture if using. Place the blueberries and mint leaves in a blender. Blend on high for 30 to 60 seconds, until uniformly combined.
2. Mix the lemonade. In a pitcher, combine the lemon juice and raw honey, stirring until the honey dissolves. Add the berry mixture if using and stir to incorporate.
3. Serve. Pour in the water and add ice if desired. Stir well to combine.
4. Storage. Best enjoyed fresh, but this lemonade can be stored in a tightly sealed container in the refrigerator for up to 3 days.

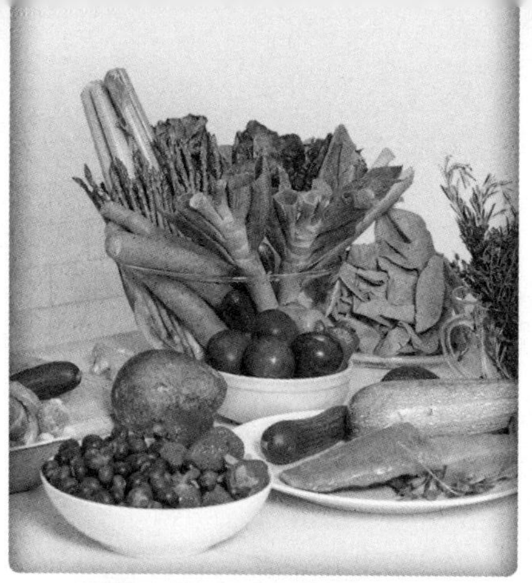

References

ACP-ASIM and BMJ Publishing Group for Evidence-Based Medicine. (1999). Review: Vitamin B6 is beneficial in the premenstrual syndrome. *BMJ Evidence-Based Medicine, 4,* 182.

Ağagündüz, D., Şahin, T. Ö., Yılmaz, B., Ekenci, K. D., Duyar Özer, Ş., & Capasso, R. (2022). Cruciferous vegetables and their bioactive metabolites: From prevention to novel therapies of colorectal cancer. *Evidence-Based Complementary and Alternative Medicine: eCAM, 2022*, 1534083. https://doi.org/10.1155/2022/1534083

Age-Related Eye Disease Study Research Group. (2001). A randomized, placebo-controlled, clinical trial of high-dose supplementation with vitamins C and E, beta carotene, and zinc for age-related macular degeneration and vision loss: AREDS Report No. 8. *Archives of Ophthalmology, 119*(10), 1417–1436. doi:10.1001/archopht.119.10.1417

Al Damen, L., Stockton, A., & Al-Dujaili, E. A. S. (2018). Effects on cognition of berry, pomegranate, grape, and biophenols:

A general review. *The Journal of Prevention of Alzheimer's Disease (JPAD)*. https://doi.org/10.14283/jpad.2018.21

Al-Kaisy, Q. H., Al-Saadi, J. S., Al-Rikabi, A. K. J., Altemimi, A. B., Hesarinejad, M. A., & Abedelmaksoud, T. G. (2023). Exploring the health benefits and functional properties of goat milk proteins. *Food Science & Nutrition, 11*(10), 5641–5656. https://doi.org/10.1002/fsn3.3531

Añazco, C., Ojeda, P. G., & Guerrero-Wyss, M. (2023). Common beans as a source of amino acids and cofactors for collagen biosynthesis. *Nutrients, 15*(21), 4561. https://doi.org/10.3390/nu15214561

Anderson, R. A., Cheng, N., Bryden, N. A., Polansky, M. M., Cheng, N., Chi, J., & Feng, J. (1997). Elevated intakes of supplemental chromium improve glucose and insulin variables in individuals with type 2 diabetes. *Diabetes, 46*(11), 1786–1791. https://doi.org/10.2337/diab.46.11.1786

Archdall, R. (2023, January 21). Water, thoughts and emotions: The effect on water. My Water Filter. https://mywaterfilter.com.au/blogs/learning/how-water-responds-to-thoughts-and-emotions

Avant Interventional Psychiatry. (n.d.). The connection between the gut and mental health. *Cell Host & Microbe*. https://www.avantpsychiatry.com/connection-between-gut-and-mental-health

Babaei, F., Mirzababaei, M., & Nassiri-Asl, M. (2018). Quercetin in food: Possible mechanisms of its effect on memory. *Journal of Food Science, 83*(9), 2280–2287. https://doi.org/10.1111/1750-3841.14317

Banskota, S., Ghia, J.-E., & Khan, W. I. (2018). Serotonin in the gut: Blessing or a curse? *Biochimica et Biophysica Acta (BBA)—Molecular Basis of Disease, 1864*(10), 1499–1508. https://doi.org/10.1016/j.biochi.2018.06.008

Baskaran, K., Kizar Ahamath, B., Radha Shanmugasundaram, K., & Shanmugasundaram, E. R. (1990). Antidiabetic effect of a leaf extract from Gymnema sylvestre in non-insulin-dependent diabetes mellitus patients. *Journal of Ethnopharmacology, 30*(3), 295–300. https://doi.org/10.1016/0378-8741(90)90108-6

Basnet, J., Eissa, M. A., Yanes Cardozo, L. L., Romero, D. G., & Rezq, S. (2024). Impact of probiotics and prebiotics on gut microbiome and hormonal regulation. *Gastrointestinal Disorders, 6*(4), 801–815. https://doi.org/10.3390/gidisord6040056

Batista da Silva Galdino, A., do Nascimento Rangel, A. H., Buttar, H. S., Sales Lima Nascimento, M., Cristina Gavioli, E., Oliveira, R. de P., . . . Anaya, K. (2021). Bovine colostrum: Benefits for the human respiratory system and potential contributions for clinical management of COVID-19. *Food and Agricultural Immunology, 32*(1), 143–162. https://doi.org/10.1080/09540105.2021.1892594

Bauer, J., Biolo, G., Cederholm, T. M., Cesari, M., Cruz-Jentoft, A. J., Morley, J. E., Phillips, S., Sieber, C., Stehle, P., Teta, D., Visvanathan, R., Volpi, E., Boirie, Y. (2013). Evidence-based recommendations for optimal dietary protein intake in older people: A position paper from the prot-age study group. *Journal of the American Medical Directors Association, 14*(8), 542–559. https://doi.org/10.1016/j.jamda.2013.05.021

Bemark, M., Pitcher, M. J., Dionisi, C., & Spencer, J. (2024). Gut-associated lymphoid tissue: A microbiota-driven hub of B cell immunity. *Trends in Immunology, 45*(3), 211–223. https://doi.org/10.1016/j.it.2024.01.006

Berkheiser, K. (2019, November 21). What's the difference between tofu and tempeh? Healthline. https://www.healthline.com/nutrition/tempeh-vs-tofu

Berman, A. Y., Motechin, R. A., Wiesenfeld, M. Y., & Holz, M. K. (2017). The therapeutic potential of resveratrol: A review of clinical trials. *NPJ Precision Oncology, 1,* 35. https://doi.org/10.1038/s41698-017-0038-6

Berrazaga, I., Micard, V., Gueugneau, M., & Walrand, S. (2019). The role of the anabolic properties of plant- versus animal-based protein sources in supporting muscle mass maintenance: A critical review. *Nutrients, 11*(8), 1825. https://doi.org/10.3390/nu11081825

Bisdee, J. T., Garlick, P. J., & James, W. P. T. (1989). Metabolic changes during the menstrual cycle. *British Journal of Nutrition 61,* 641–650. https://www.cambridge.org/core/services/aop-cambridge-core/content/view/CCA85CDEDD3513EBCAE8158637058E95/S0007114589000711a.pdf/metabolic-changes-during-the-menstrual-cycle.pdf

Blumberg, J. B., Camesano, T. A., Cassidy, A., Kris-Etherton, P., Howell, A., Manach, C., Ostertag, L. M., Sies, H., Skulas-Ray, A., & Vita, J. A. (2013). Cranberries and their bioactive constituents in human health. *Advances in Nutrition (Bethesda, Md.), 4*(6), 618–632. https://doi.org/10.3945/an.113.004473

Bookheimer, S. Y., Renner, B. A., Ekstrom, A., Li, Z., Henning, S. M., Brown, J. A., Jones, M., Moody, T., & Small, G. W. (2013). Pomegranate juice augments memory and FMRI activity in middle-aged and older adults with mild memory complaints. *Evidence-Based Complementary and Alternative Medicine: eCAM, 2013*, 946298. https://doi.org/10.1155/2013/946298

Borbolis, F., Mytilinaiou, E., & Palikaras, K. (2023). The crosstalk between microbiome and mitochondrial homeostasis in neurodegeneration. *Cells, 12*(3), 429. https://doi.org/10.3390/cells12030429

Borgeraas, H., Johnson, L. K., Skattebu, J., Hertel, J. K., & Hjelmesaeth, J. (2018). Effects of probiotics on body weight, body mass index, fat mass and fat percentage in subjects with overweight or obesity: A systematic review and meta-analysis of randomized controlled trials. *Obesity Reviews: An Official Journal of the International Association for the Study of Obesity, 19*(2), 219–232. https://doi.org/10.1111/obr.12626

Boulangé, C. L., Neves, A. L., Chilloux, J., et al. (2016). Impact of the gut microbiota on inflammation, obesity, and metabolic disease. *Genome Medicine, 8,* 42. https://doi.org/10.1186/s13073-016-0303-2

Braaten, J. T., Wood, P. J., Scott, F. W., Wolynetz, M. S., Lowe, M. K., Bradley-White, P., & Collins, M. W. (1994). Oat beta-glucan reduces blood cholesterol concentration in hypercholesterolemic subjects. *European Journal of Clinical Nutrition, 48*(7), 465–474.

Brayden, D. J., & Walsh, E. (2014). Efficacious intestinal permeation enhancement induced by the sodium salt of 10-undecylenic acid, a medium chain fatty acid derivative. *The AAPS Journal, 16*(5), 1064–1076. https://doi.org/10.1208/s12248-014-9634-3

Buettner, D., & Skemp, S. (2016). Blue zones: Lessons from the world's longest lived. *American Journal of Lifestyle Medicine, 10*(5), 318–321. https://doi.org/10.1177/1559827616637066

Burkhart, A. (2024). Histamine intolerance: Are foods causing histamine intolerance symptoms? Histamine Intolerance: Symptoms, Diet & Treatment. https://theceliacmd.com/histamine-intolerance-symptoms-diet-treatment/

Carbone, J. W., & Pasiakos, S. M. (2019). Dietary protein and muscle mass: Translating science to application and health benefit. *Nutrients, 11*(5), 1136. https://doi.org/10.3390/nu11051136

Carter, D. A., Blair, S. E., Cokcetin, N. N., Bouzo, D., Brooks, P., Schothauer, R., & Harry, E. J. (2016). Therapeutic manuka honey: No longer so alternative. *Frontiers in Microbiology, 7,* 569. https://doi.org/10.3389/fmicb.2016.00569

Chae, Y., & Lee, I. S. (2023). Central regulation of eating behaviors in humans: Evidence from functional neuroimaging studies. *Nutrients, 15*(13), 3010. https://doi.org/10.3390/nu15133010

Champion, C. (2024, July 23). Patients taking weight loss medications require proper nutrition. UCLA Health. https://www.uclahealth.org/news/article/patients-taking-weight-loss-medications-require-proper

Chausmer, A. B. (1998). Zinc, insulin and diabetes. *Journal of the American College of Nutrition, 17*(2), 109–115. https://doi.org/10.1080/07315724.1998.10718735\

Chen, P. E., Liu, C. Y., Chien, W. H., Chien, C. W., & Tung, T. H. (2019). Effectiveness of cherries in reducing uric acid and gout: A systematic review. *Evidence-Based Complementary and Alternative Medicine: eCAM, 2019*, 9896757. https://doi.org/10.1155/2019/9896757

Chen, Y., Xu, J., & Chen, Y. (2021). Regulation of neurotransmitters by the gut microbiota and effects on cognition in neurological disorders. *Nutrients, 13*(6), 2099. https://doi.org/10.3390/nu13062099

Cheng, F. W., Ford, N. A., & Taylor, M. K. (2021). US older adults that consume avocado or guacamole have better cognition than non-consumers: National Health and Nutrition Examination Survey 2011–2014. *Frontiers in Nutrition, 8,* 746453. https://doi.org/10.3389/fnut.2021.746453

Cheng, P., Neugaard, B., Foulis, P., & Conlin, P. R. (2011). Hemoglobin A1c as a predictor of incident diabetes. *Diabetes Care, 34*(3), 610–615. https://doi.org/10.2337/dc10-0625

Chinnadurai, K., Kanwal, H. K., Tyagi, A. K., Stanton, C., & Ross, P. (2013). High-conjugated linoleic acid-enriched ghee (clarified butter) increases the antioxidant and antiatherogenic potency in female Wistar rats. *Lipids in Health and Disease, 12,* 121. https://doi.org/10.1186/1476-511X-12-121

Chong, P. P., Chin, V. K., Looi, C. Y., Wong, W. F., Madhavan, P., & Yong, V. C. (2021). The microbiome and irritable bowel syndrome: A review of the pathophysiology, current research, and future therapy updated. *Frontiers in Medicine, 8,* 738502. https://doi.org/10.3389/fmed.2021.738502

Clapp, M., Aurora, N., Herrera, L., Bhatia, M., Wilen, E., & Wakefield, S. (2017). Gut microbiota's effect on mental health: The gut-brain axis. *Clinics and Practice, 7*(4), 987. https://doi.org/10.4081/cp.2017.987

Clemente-Suárez, V. J., Beltrán-Velasco, A. I., Redondo-Flórez, L., Martín-Rodríguez, A., & Tornero-Aguilera, J. F. (2023). Global impacts of Western diet and its effects on metabolism and health: A narrative review. *Nutrients, 15*(12), 2749. https://doi.org/10.3390/nu15122749

Cleveland Clinic. (n.d.). Low FODMAP diet. https://my.clevelandclinic.org/health/treatments/22466-low-fodmap-diet

Cömert, E. D., Mogol, B. A., & Gökmen, V. (2019). Relationship between color and antioxidant capacity of fruits and vegetables. *Current Research in Food Science, 2,* 1–10. https://doi.org/10.1016/j.crfs.2019.11.001

Conversation, The. (2024, September 4). How the health of your gut microbiome can affect your skin. https://theconversation.com/how-the-health-of-your-gut-microbiome-can-affect-your-skin-230286

Covarrubias, A. J., Perrone, R., Grozio, A., & Verdin, E. (2021). NAD+ metabolism and its roles in cellular processes during ageing. Nature reviews. *Molecular Cell Biology, 22*(2), 119–141. https://doi.org/10.1038/s41580-020-00313-x

Damián-Medina, K., Milenkovic, D., Salinas-Moreno, Y., Corral-Jara, K. F., Figueroa-Yáñez, L., Marino-Marmolejo, E., & Lugo-Cervantes, E. (2022). Anthocyanin-rich extract from black beans exerts anti-diabetic effects in rats through a multi-genomic mode of action in adipose tissue. *Frontiers in Nutrition, 9,* 1019259. https://doi.org/10.3389/fnut.2022.1019259

de Wouters d'Oplinter, A., Huwart, S. J. P., Cani, P. D., & Everard, A. (2022). Gut microbes and food reward: From the gut to the brain. *Frontiers in Neuroscience, 16,* article 947240. https://doi.org/10.3389/fnins.2022.947240

Docherty, S., Doughty, F. L., & Smith, E. F. (2023). The acute and chronic effects of lion's mane mushroom supplementation on cognitive function, stress and mood in young adults: A double-blind, parallel groups, pilot study. *Nutrients, 15*(22), 4842. https://doi.org/10.3390/nu15224842

Ehren, J., Morón, B., Martin, E., Bethune, M. T., Gray, G. M., & Khosla, C. (2009). A food-grade enzyme preparation with modest gluten detoxification properties. *PLOS One, 4*(7), e6313. https://doi.org/10.1371/journal.pone.0006313

Ellis, S. R., Nguyen, M., Vaughn, A. R., Notay, M., Burney, W. A., Sandhu, S., & Sivamani, R. K. (2019). The skin and gut microbiome and its role in common dermatologic conditions. *Microorganisms, 7*(11), 550. https://doi.org/10.3390/microorganisms7110550

Evans, J. L., & Goldfine, I. D. (2000). Alpha-lipoic acid: A multifunctional antioxidant that improves insulin sensitivity in patients with type 2 diabetes. *Diabetes Technology & Therapeutics, 2*(3), 401–413. https://doi.org/10.1089/15209150050194279

EWG's Shopper's Guide to Pesticides in Produce. (2024). *EWG's shopper's guide: The 2024 Dirty Dozen.* https://www.ewg.org/foodnews/dirty-dozen.php

Fagundes, C. P., Bennett, J. M., Derry, H. M., & Kiecolt-Glaser, J. K. (2011). Relationships and inflammation across the lifespan: Social developmental pathways to disease. *Social and Personality Psychology Compass, 5*(11), 891–903. https://doi.org/10.1111/j.1751-9004.2011.00392.x

Fahey, J. W., Holtzclaw, W. D., Wehage, S. L., Wade, K. L., Stephenson, K. K., & Talalay, P. (2015). Sulforaphane bioavailability from glucoraphanin-rich broccoli: Control by active endogenous myrosinase. *PLOS One, 10*(11), e0140963. https://doi.org/10.1371/journal.pone.0140963

Fahey, J. W., Zhang, Y., & Talalay, P. (1997). Broccoli sprouts: An exceptionally rich source of inducers of enzymes that protect against chemical carcinogens. *Proceedings of the National Academy of Sciences of the United States of America, 94*(19), 10367–10372. https://doi.org/10.1073/pnas.94.19.10367

Farris, P. K., Engelman, D., Day, D., Hazan, A., & Raymond, I. (2023). Natural hair supplements: Trends and myths untangled. *Journal of Clinical and Aesthetic Dermatology, 16*(1 Suppl 1), S4–S11.

Fasano, A. (2012). Leaky gut and autoimmune diseases. *Clinical Reviews in Allergy & Immunology, 42*(1), 71–78. https://doi.org/10.1007/s12016-011-8291-x

Fisher, M., & Yang, L. X. (2002). Anticancer effects and mechanisms of polysaccharide-K (PSK): Implications of cancer immunotherapy. *Anticancer Research, 22*(3), 1737–1754.

Frazie, M. D., Kim, M. J., & Ku, K. M. (2017). Health-promoting phytochemicals from 11 mustard cultivars at baby leaf and mature stages. *Molecules (Basel, Switzerland), 22*(10), 1749. https://doi.org/10.3390/molecules22101749

Frey, M. (2024, June 6). Beef liver nutrition facts and health benefits. VeryWell. https://www.verywellfit.com/beef-liver-nutrition-facts-and-health-benefits-5025125

Friedman, M. (2015). Chemistry, nutrition, and health-promoting properties of Hericium erinaceus (lion's mane) mushroom fruiting bodies and mycelia and their bioactive compounds. *Journal of Agricultural and Food Chemistry, 63*(32), 7108–7123. https://doi.org/10.1021/acs.jafc.5b02914

Gault, Z. (2024, January 11). The collagen boost: Exploring the role of vitamin C in collagen synthesis. For Youth. https://foryouth.co/blogs/magazine/collagen-boost-vitamin-c-in-collagen-synthesis

Gemesi, K., Holzmann, S. L., Kaiser, B. et al. (2022). Stress eating: An online survey of eating behaviours, comfort foods, and healthy food substitutes in German adults. *BMC Public Health, 22,* 391. https://doi.org/10.1186/s12889-022-12787-9

Giménez-Bastida, J. A., & Zieliński, H. (2015). Buckwheat as a functional food and its effects on health. *Journal of Agricultural and Food Chemistry, 63*(36), 7896–7913. https://doi.org/10.1021/acs.jafc.5b02498

Glazier, E. M., & Ko, E. (2021, October 1). Circadian diet another form of intermittent fasting. UCLA Health. https://www.uclahealth.org/news/article/circadian-diet-another-form-of-intermittent-fasting

Greenhill, C. (2014). Not so sweet: Artificial sweeteners can cause glucose intolerance by affecting the gut microbiota. *Nature Reviews Endocrinology, 10,* 637. https://doi.org/10.1038/nrendo.2014.167

Griffin, R. M. (2023, August 1). Coenzyme Q10 (CoQ10). https://www.webmd.com/diet/supplement-guide-coenzymeq10-coq10

Gocki, J., & Bartuzi, Z. (2016). Role of immunoglobulin G antibodies in diagnosis of food allergy. *Postepy Dermatologii i Alergologii, 33*(4), 253–256. https://doi.org/10.5114/ada.2016.61600

Gopukumar, K., Thanawala, S., Somepalli, V., Rao, T. S. S., Thamatam, V. B., & Chauhan, S. (2021). Efficacy and safety of ashwagandha root extract on cognitive functions in healthy, stressed adults: A randomized, double-blind, placebo-controlled study. *Evidence-Based Complementary and Alternative Medicine: eCAM, 2021,* 8254344. https://doi.org/10.1155/2021/8254344

Guerrero-Romero, F., & Rodríguez-Morán, M. (2002). Low serum magnesium levels and metabolic syndrome. *Acta diabetologica, 39*(4), 209–213. https://doi.org/10.1007/s005920200036

Guinter, M. A., Sandler, D. P., McLain, A. C., Merchant, A. T., & Steck, S. E. (2018). An estrogen-related dietary pattern and postmenopausal breast cancer risk in a cohort of women with a family history of breast cancer. *Cancer Epidemiology, Biomarkers & Prevention: A Publication of the American Association for Cancer Research, Cosponsored by the American Society of Preventive Oncology, 27*(10), 1223–1226. https://doi.org/10.1158/1055-9965.EPI-18-0514

Habeeb, F., Shakir, E., Bradbury, F., Cameron, P., Taravati, M. R., Drummond, A. J., Gray, A. I., & Ferro, V. A. (2007). Screening methods used to determine the anti-microbial properties of aloe vera inner gel. *Methods (San Diego, Calif.), 42*(4), 315–320. https://doi.org/10.1016/j.ymeth.2007.03.004

Hackney, A. C. (2021). Menstrual cycle hormonal changes and energy substrate metabolism in exercising women: A perspective. *International Journal of Environmental Research and Public Health, 18*(19), 10024. https://doi.org/10.3390/ijerph181910024

Hakansson, A., & Molin, G. (2011). Gut microbiota and inflammation. *Nutrients, 3*(6), 637–682. https://doi.org/10.3390/nu3060637

Hall, K. D., & Kahan, S. (2018). Maintenance of lost weight and long-term management of obesity. *The Medical Clinics of North America, 102*(1), 183–197. https://doi.org/10.1016/j.mcna.2017.08.012

Hawkins, J., Baker, C., Cherry, L., & Dunne, E. (2019). Black elderberry (Sambucus nigra) supplementation effectively treats upper respiratory symptoms: A meta-analysis of randomized, controlled clinical trials. *Complementary Therapies in Medicine, 42,* 361–365. https://doi.org/10.1016/j.ctim.2018.12.004

Hayashida, H., Shimura, M., Sugama, K., & Kanda, K. (2016). Exercise-induced inflammation during different phases of the menstrual cycle. *Journal of Physiotherapy & Physical Rehabilitation, 1*(4), article 1000121. https://doi.org/10.4172/2573-0312.1000121

Heart Health. (2019, July 1). New insights about inflammation. Harvard Health Publishing. https://www.health.harvard.edu/heart-health/new-insights-about-inflammation

Hensrud, D. (n.d.). Nutrition and healthy eating. Mayo Clinic. https://www.mayoclinic.org/healthy-lifestyle/nutrition-and-healthy-eating/expert-answers/coffee-and-health/faq-20058339

Herdman, R. (n.d.). PMS is helped by 5-HTP. Pacific Center for Naturopathic Medicine. https://doctorherdmanclinic.com/resources/articles/womens-health/pms-5-htp/

Hess, J. M., Stephensen, C. B., Kratz, M., & Bolling, B. W. (2021). Exploring the links between diet and inflammation: Dairy foods as case studies. *Advances in Nutrition (Bethesda, Md.), 12*(Suppl 1), 1S–13S. https://doi.org/10.1093/advances/nmab108

Higdon, J. V., Delage, B., Williams, D. E., & Dashwood, R. H. (2007). Cruciferous vegetables and human cancer risk: Epidemiologic evidence and mechanistic basis. *Pharmacological Research, 55*(3), 224–236. https://doi.org/10.1016/j.phrs.2007.01.009

Hoes, M. F., Grote Beverborg, N., Kijlstra, J. D., Kuipers, J., Swinkels, D. W., Giepmans, B. N. G., Rodenburg, R. J., van Veldhuisen, D. J., de Boer, R. A., & van der Meer, P. (2018). Iron deficiency impairs contractility of human cardiomyocytes through decreased mitochondrial function. *European Journal of Heart Failure, 20*(5), 910–919. https://doi.org/10.1002/ejhf.1154

Holtzman, B., & Ackerman, K. E. (2021). Recommendations and nutritional considerations for female athletes: Health and performance. *Sports Medicine (Auckland, N.Z.), 51*(Suppl 1), 43–57. https://doi.org/10.1007/s40279-021-01508-8

Horn, A. J., & Carter, C. S. (2021). Love and longevity: A social dependency hypothesis. *Comprehensive Psychoneuroendocrinology, 8*, 100088. https://doi.org/10.1016/j.cpnec.2021.100088

Howatson, G., Bell, P. G., Tallent, J., Middleton, B., McHugh, M. P., & Ellis, J. (2012). Effect of tart cherry juice (Prunus cerasus) on melatonin levels and enhanced sleep quality. *European Journal of Nutrition, 51*(8), 909–916. https://doi.org/10.1007/s00394-011-0263-7

Howes, L. (Host). (2018, March 19). Dr. Mark Hyman: Heal your body with food. Lewis Howes (podcast). https://lewishowes.com/podcast/i-dr-mark-.hyman-heal-your-body-with-food/

Hromatko, I., & Mikac, U. (2023). A mid-cycle rise in positive and drop in negative moods among healthy young women: A pilot study. *Brain Sciences, 13*(1), 105. https://doi.org/10.3390/brainsci13010105

Hu, S., Ding, Q., Zhang, W., Kang, M., Ma, J., & Zhao, L. (2023). Gut microbial beta-glucuronidase: A vital regulator in female estrogen metabolism. *Gut Microbes, 15*(1), 2236749. https://doi.org/10.1080/19490976.2023.2236749

Huang, H., Jia, C., Chen, X., Zhang, L., Jiang, Y., Meng, X., & Liu, X. (2024). Progress in research on the effects of quinoa (Chenopodium quinoa) bioactive compounds and products on intestinal flora. *Frontiers in Nutrition, 11,* 1308384. https://doi.org/10.3389/fnut.2024.1308384

Husain, M., Zaigham, M.,–Hamiduddin, Wadud, A., & Ali, M. A. (2021). A review on pharmacological and phytochemical profile of khatmi (Althaea officinalis Linn.): An important mucilaginous plant and its utilization in Unani system of medicine. *International Journal of Research in Ayurveda and Pharmacy, 12*, 376–382. https://doi.org/10.7897/2277-4343.120376.

Hussain, J., & Cohen, M. (2018). Clinical effects of regular dry sauna bathing: A systematic review. *Evidence-Based Complementary and Alternative Medicine: eCAM, 2018,* 1857413. https://doi.org/10.1155/2018/1857413

Ispas, S., Tuta, L. A., Botnarciuc, M., Ispas, V., Staicovici, S., Ali, S., Nelson-Twakor, A., Cojocaru, C., Herlo, A., & Petcu, A. (2023). Metabolic disorders, the microbiome as an endocrine organ, and their relations with obesity: A literature review. *Journal of Personalized Medicine, 13*(11), 1602. https://doi.org/10.3390/jpm13111602

Jenkins, T. A., Nguyen, J. C., Polglaze, K. E., & Bertrand, P. P. (2016). Influence of tryptophan and serotonin on mood and cognition with a possible role of the gut-brain axis. *Nutrients, 8*(1), 56. https://doi.org/10.3390/nu8010056

Jianqin, S., Leiming, X., Lu, X., et al. (2015). Effects of milk containing only A2 beta casein versus milk containing both A1 and A2 beta casein proteins on gastrointestinal physiology, symptoms of discomfort, and cognitive behavior of people with self-reported intolerance to traditional cows' milk. *Nutrition Journal, 15,* 35 https://doi.org/10.1186/s12937-016-0147-z

Johnson, E. J. (2014). Role of lutein and zeaxanthin in visual and cognitive function throughout the lifespan. *Nutrition Reviews, 72*(9), 605–612. https://doi.org/10.1111/nure.12133

Juhl, C. R., Bergholdt, H. K. M., Miller, I. M., Jemec, G. B. E., Kanters, J. K., & Ellervik, C. (2018). Dairy intake and acne vulgaris: A systematic review and meta-analysis of 78,529 children, adolescents, and young adults. *Nutrients, 10*(8), 1049. https://doi.org/10.3390/nu10081049

Kanetkar, P., Singhal, R., & Kamat, M. (2007). Gymnema sylvestre: A memoir. *Journal of Clinical Biochemistry and Nutrition, 41*(2), 77–81. https://doi.org/10.3164/jcbn.2007010

Kato, H., Suzuki, K., Bannai, M., & Moore, D. R. (2016). Protein requirements are elevated in endurance athletes after exercise as determined by the indicator amino acid oxidation method. *PLOS One, 11*(6), e0157406. https://doi.org/10.1371/journal.pone.0157406

Keller, J. L., Housh, T. J., Hill, E. C., Smith, C. M., Schmidt, R. J., & Johnson, G. O. (2019). The effects of Shilajit supplementation on fatigue-induced decreases in muscular strength and serum hydroxyproline levels. *Journal of the International Society of Sports Nutrition, 16*(1), 3. https://doi.org/10.1186/s12970-019-0270-2

Kennedy, D. O. (2016). B Vitamins and the brain: Mechanisms, dose and efficacy—a review. *Nutrients, 8*(2), 68. https://doi.org/10.3390/nu8020068

Khan, A., Safdar, M., Khan, M. M. A., Khattak, K. N., & Anderson, R. A. (2003). Cinnamon improves glucose and lipids of people with type 2 diabetes. *Diabetes Care, 26*(12), 3215–3218. https://doi.org/10.2337/diacare.26.12.3215

Khan, F. (2024, January 21). Niacin: Boosting hair growth and scalp health. Fully Vital (podcast). https://fullyvital.com/blogs/hair-vitamins/niacin

Kim, H., Caulfield, L. E., & Rebholz, C. M. (2018). Healthy plant-based diets are associated with lower risk of all-cause mortality in US adults. *The Journal of Nutrition, 148*(4), 624–631. https://doi.org/10.1093/jn/nxy019

Kim, H. M., & Kim, J. (2013). The effects of green tea on obesity and type 2 diabetes. *Diabetes & Metabolism Journal, 37*(3), 173–175. https://doi.org/10.4093/dmj.2013.37.3.173

Kissow, J., Jacobsen, K. J., Gunnarsson, T. P., Jessen, S., & Hostrup, M. (2022). Effects of follicular and luteal phase-based menstrual cycle resistance training on muscle strength and mass. *Sports Medicine (Auckland, N.Z.), 52*(12), 2813–2819. https://doi.org/10.1007/s40279-022-01679-y

Ko, D. Y., Seo, S. M., Lee, Y. H., et al. (2024). Turning glucosinolate into allelopathic fate: Investigating allyl isothiocyanate variability and nitrile formation in eco-friendly Brassica juncea from South Korea. *Scientific Reports, 14,* 15423 https://doi.org/10.1038/s41598-024-65938-w

Kreider, R. B., & Stout, J. R. (2021). Creatine in health and disease. *Nutrients, 13*(2), 447. https://doi.org/10.3390/nu13020447

Kuan, W. H., Chen, Y. L., & Liu, C. L. (2022). Excretion of Ni, Pb, Cu, As, and Hg in sweat under two sweating conditions. *International Journal of Environmental Research and Public Health, 19*(7), 4323. https://doi.org/10.3390/ijerph19074323

Lai, Y., Masatoshi, H., Ma, Y., Guo, Y., & Zhang, B. (2022). Role of vitamin K in intestinal health. *Frontiers in Immunology, 12,* article 791565. https://doi.org/10.3389/fimmu.2021.791565

Lang, A. (2021, May 21). *6 surprising health benefits of caviar.* Healthline. https://www.healthline.com/nutrition/caviar-benefits

Lautrup, S., Sinclair, D. A., Mattson, M. P., & Fang, E. F. (2019). NAD+ in brain aging and neurodegenerative disorders. *Cell Metabolism, 30*(4), 630–655. https://doi.org/10.1016/j.cmet.2019.09.001

León-López, A., Morales-Peñaloza, A., Martínez-Juárez, V. M., Vargas-Torres, A., Zeugolis, D. I., & Aguirre-Álvarez, G. (2019). Hydrolyzed collagen-sources and applications. *Molecules (Basel, Switzerland), 24*(22), 4031. https://doi.org/10.3390/molecules24224031

Leszczyńska, J., Szczepankowska, A. K., Majak, I., Mańkowska, D., Smolińska, B., Ścieszka, S., Diowksz, A., Cukrowska, B., & Aleksandrzak-Piekarczyk, T. (2024). Reducing immunoreactivity of gluten peptides by probiotic lactic acid bacteria for dietary management of gluten-related diseases. *Nutrients, 16*(7), 976. https://doi.org/10.3390/nu16070976

Leung, L., Birtwhistle, R., Kotecha, J., Hannah, S., & Cuthbertson, S. (2009). Anti-diabetic and hypoglycaemic effects of Momordica charantia (bitter melon): A mini review. *The British Journal of Nutrition, 102*(12), 1703–1708. https://doi.org/10.1017/S0007114509992054

Li, C., Lin, J., Yang, T., & Shang, H. (2022). Green tea intake and Parkinson's disease progression: A Mendelian randomization study. *Frontiers in Nutrition, 9,* 848223. https://doi.org/10.3389/fnut.2022.848223

Li, I. C., Lee, L. Y., Tzeng, T. T., Chen, W. P., Chen, Y. P., Shiao, Y. J., & Chen, C. C. (2018, May 21). Neurohealth properties of Hericium erinaceus mycelia enriched with erinacines. *Behavioural Neurology,* 5802634. https://doi.org/10.1155/2018/5802634

Li, P., & Wu, G. (2018). Roles of dietary glycine, proline, and hydroxyproline in collagen synthesis and animal growth. *Amino Acids, 50,* 29–38. https://doi.org/10.1007/s00726-017-2490-6

Logan, A. C., & Katzman, M. (2005). Major depressive disorder: Probiotics may be an adjuvant therapy. *Medical Hypotheses, 64*(3), 533–538. https://doi.org/10.1016/j.mehy.2004.08.019

Lordan, R., Tsoupras, A., Mitra, B., & Zabetakis, I. (2018). Dairy fats and cardiovascular disease: Do we really need to be Concerned? *Foods (Basel, Switzerland), 7*(3), 29. https://doi.org/10.3390/foods7030029

Louis, S. (2024, March 26). "One of the biggest wastes of money": Suze Orman doesn't want you to eat out. Moneywise. https://moneywise.com/managing-money/budgeting/suze-orman-refuses-to-eat-out

Ludwig, D. S., & Ebbeling, C. B. (2018). The carbohydrate-insulin model of obesity: Beyond "calories in, calories out." *JAMA Internal Medicine, 178*(8), 1098–1103. https://doi.org/10.1001/jamainternmed.2018.2933

Ludwig, D. S., Willett, W. C., Volek, J. S., & Neuhouser, M. L. (2018). Dietary fat: From foe to friend? *Science (New York), 362*(6416), 764–770. https://doi.org/10.1126/science.aau2096

Madison, A., & Kiecolt-Glaser, J. K. (2019). Stress, depression, diet, and the gut microbiota: Human-bacteria interactions at the core of psychoneuroimmunology and nutrition. *Current Opinion in Behavioral Sciences, 28,* 105–110. https://doi.org/10.1016/j.cobeha.2019.01.011

Mahmud, M. R., Akter, S., Tamanna, S. K., Mazumder, L., Esti, I. Z., Banerjee, S., Akter, S., Hasan, M. R., Acharjee, M., Hossain, M. S., & Pirttilä, A. M. (2022). Impact of gut microbiome on skin health:

Gut-skin axis observed through the lenses of therapeutics and skin diseases. *Gut Microbes, 14*(1), 2096995. https://doi.org/10.1080/19490976.2022.2096995

Makki, K., Deehan, E. C., Walter, J., & Bäckhed, F. (2018). The impact of dietary fiber on gut microbiota in host health and disease. *Cell Host & Microbe, 23*(6), 705–715. https://doi.org/10.1016/j.chom.2018.05.012

Mansfield, R. (2023, September 27). Could you eat 30 plant-based foods a week? World Cancer Research Fund. https://www.wcrf.org/about-us/news-and-blogs/could-you-eat-30-plant-based-foods-each-week/

Marco, M. L., Heeney, D., Binda, S., Cifelli, C. J., Cotter, P. D., Foligné, B., Gänzle, M., Kort, R., Pasin, G., Pihlanto, A., Smid, E. J., & Hutkins, R. (2017). Health benefits of fermented foods: Microbiota and beyond. *Current Opinion in Biotechnology, 44*, 94–102. https://doi.org/10.1016/j.copbio.2016.11.010

Mariotti, F., & Gardner, C. D. (2019). Dietary protein and amino acids in vegetarian diets: A review. *Nutrients, 11*(11), 2661. https://doi.org/10.3390/nu11112661

Markofski, M. M., & Braun, W. A. (2014). Influence of menstrual cycle on indices of contraction-induced muscle damage. *Journal of Strength and Conditioning Research, 28*(9), 2649–2656. https://doi.org/10.1519/JSC.0000000000000429

Martínez, Y., Li, X., Liu, G., Bin, P., Yan, W., Más, D., Valdivié, M., Hu, C. A., Ren, W., & Yin, Y. (2017). The role of methionine on metabolism, oxidative stress, and diseases. *Amino Acids, 49*(12), 2091–2098. https://doi.org/10.1007/s00726-017-2494-2

Masterman, S. (2022, April 13). Reishi mushroom: Queen of the mushroom kingdom. Rheal Superfoods. https://rhealsuperfoods.com/blogs/news/health-benefits-of-reishi-mushroom

Maughan, R. J., & Shirreffs, S. M. (2008). Development of individual hydration strategies for athletes. *International Journal of Sport Nutrition and Exercise Metabolism, 18*(5), 457–472. https://doi.org/10.1123/ijsnem.18.5.457

McCarthy, D., & Berg, A. (2021). Weight loss strategies and the risk of skeletal muscle mass loss. *Nutrients, 13*(7), 2473. https://doi.org/10.3390/nu13072473

McDonald, D., Hyde, E., Debelius, J. W., Morton, J. T., Gonzalez, A., Ackermann, G., Aksenov, A. A., Behsaz, B., Brennan, C., Chen, Y., DeRight Goldasich, L., Dorrestein, P. C., Dunn, R. R., Fahimipour, A. K., Gaffney, J., Gilbert, J. A., Gogul, G., Green, J. L., Hugenholtz, P., Humphrey, G., . . . Knight, R. (2018). American gut: An open platform for citizen science microbiome research. *mSystems, 3*(3), e00031–18. https://doi.org/10.1128/mSystems.00031-18

Mirończuk-Chodakowska, I., Kujawowicz, K., & Witkowska, A. M. (2021). Beta-glucans from fungi: Biological and health-promoting potential in the COVID-19 pandemic era. *Nutrients, 13*(11), 3960. https://doi.org/10.3390/nu13113960

Moghaddam, E., Vogt, J. A., & Wolever, T. M. (2006). The effects of fat and protein on glycemic responses in nondiabetic humans vary with waist circumference, fasting plasma insulin, and dietary fiber intake. *The Journal of Nutrition, 136*(10), 2506–2511. https://doi.org/10.1093/jn/136.10.2506

Mori, K., Inatomi, S., Ouchi, K., Azumi, Y., & Tuchida, T. (2009). Improving effects of the mushroom Yamabushitake (Hericium erinaceus) on mild cognitive impairment: A double-blind placebo-controlled clinical trial. *Phytotherapy Research: PTR, 23*(3), 367–372. https://doi.org/10.1002/ptr.2634

Mozaffarian, D. (2016). Dietary and policy priorities for cardiovascular disease, diabetes, and obesity: A comprehensive review. *Circulation, 133*(2), 187–225. https://doi.org/10.1161/CIRCULATIONAHA.115.018585

———. (2019). Dairy foods, obesity, and metabolic health: The role of the food matrix compared with single nutrients. *Advances in Nutrition (Bethesda, Md.), 10*(5), 917S–923S. https://doi.org/10.1093/advances/nmz053

Multescu, M., Culetu, A., & Susman, I. E. (2024). Screening of the nutritional properties, bioactive components, and antioxidant properties in legumes. *Foods, 13*(22), 3528. https://doi.org/10.3390/foods13223528

National Institutes of Health. (n.d.). Vitamin A and carotenoids. U.S. Department of Health and Human Services. https://ods.od.nih.gov/factsheets/VitaminA-Consumer/

———. (n.d.). Vitamin B_{12}. U.S. Department of Health and Human Services. https://ods.od.nih.gov/factsheets/VitaminB12-Consumer/

Neeland, I. J., Linge, J., & Birkenfeld, A. L. (2024). Changes in lean body mass with glucagon-like peptide-1-based therapies and mitigation strategies. *Diabetes, Obesity & Metabolism, 26*(Suppl 4), 16–27. https://doi.org/10.1111/dom.15728

Negro, M., Giardina, S., Marzani, B., & Marzatico, F. (2008). Branched-chain amino acid supplementation does not enhance athletic performance but affects muscle recovery and the immune system. *The Journal of Sports Medicine and Physical Fitness, 48*(3), 347–351.

Nehlig, A. (2022). Effects of coffee on the gastro-intestinal tract: A narrative review and literature update. *Nutrients, 14*(2), 399. https://doi.org/10.3390/nu14020399

Nutrition Source, The. (n.d.). Nutrition and immunity. Harvard T.H. Chan School of Public Health. https://nutritionsource.hsph.harvard.edu/nutrition-and-immunity/

Opara, E. I., & Chohan, M. (2014). Culinary herbs and spices: Their bioactive properties, the contribution of polyphenols and the challenges in deducing their true health benefits. *International Journal of Molecular Sciences, 15*(10), 19183–19202. https://doi.org/10.3390/ijms151019183

O'Reilly, G. A., Cook, L., Spruijt-Metz, D., & Black, D. S. (2014). Mindfulness-based interventions for obesity-related eating behaviours: A literature review. *Obesity Reviews: An Official Journal of the International Association for the Study of Obesity, 15*(6), 453–461. https://doi.org/10.1111/obr.12156

Park, Y. W., & Nam, M. S. (2015). Bioactive peptides in milk and dairy products: A review. *Korean Journal for Food Science of Animal Resources, 35*(6), 831–840. https://doi.org/10.5851/kosfa.2015.35.6.831

Parolo, S., Lacroix, S., Kaput, J., & Scott-Boyer, M. P. (2017). Ancestors' dietary patterns and environments could drive positive selection in genes involved in micronutrient metabolism: The case of cofactor transporters. *Genes & Nutrition, 12,* 28. https://doi.org/10.1186/s12263-017-0579-x

Pashaei, K. H. A., Irankhah, K., Namkhah, Z., et al. (2024). Edible mushrooms as an alternative to animal proteins for having a more sustainable diet: A review. *Journal of Health, Population and Nutrition 43,* 205. https://doi.org/10.1186/s41043-024-00701-5

Pathan, S., & Siddiqui, R. A. (2022). Nutritional composition and bioactive components in quinoa (Chenopodium quinoa Willd.) greens: A review. *Nutrients, 14*(3), 558. https://doi.org/10.3390/nu14030558

PDQ Integrative, Alternative, and Complementary Therapies Editorial Board. (2017, March 2). Medicinal mushrooms (PDQ). National Library of Medicine. https://www.ncbi.nlm.nih.gov/books/NBK424937/

Pelc, C. (2022, July 20). Leaky gut and autoimmune disorders: Dormant "bad" gut bacteria may be key. *Medical News Today*. https://www.medicalnewstoday.com/articles/leaky-gut-and-autoimmune-disorders-dormant-bad-gut-bacteria-may-be-key

PennState. (2010, July 20). Research shows eggs from pastured chickens may be more nutritious. https://www.psu.edu/news/agricultural-sciences/story/research-shows-eggs-pastured-chickens-may-be-more-nutritious

Physiopedia. (n.d.). Gut-brain axis (GBA). https://www.physio-pedia.com/Gut_Brain_Axis_(GBA)

———. (n.d.). Vagus nerve. https://www.physio-pedia.com/Vagus_Nerve

Queiroz, K. daS., de Oliveira, A. C., Helbig, E., Reis, S. M., & Carraro, F. (2002). Soaking the common bean in a domestic preparation reduced the contents of raffinose-type oligosaccharides but did not interfere with nutritive value. *Journal of Nutritional Science and Vitaminology, 48*(4), 283–289. https://doi.org/10.3177/jnsv.48.283

Redford, K. E., & Abbott, G. W. (2020). The ubiquitous flavonoid quercetin is an atypical KCNQ potassium channel activator. *Communications Biology, 3*(1), 356. https://doi.org/10.1038/s42003-020-1089-8

Rineau, E., Gueguen, N., Procaccio, V., Geneviève, F., Reynier, P., Henrion, D., & Lasocki, S. (2021). Iron deficiency without anemia decreases physical endurance and mitochondrial complex I activity of oxidative skeletal muscle in the mouse. *Nutrients, 13*(4), 1056. https://doi.org/10.3390/nu13041056

Romero-Moraleda, B., Coso, J. D., Gutiérrez-Hellín, J., Ruiz-Moreno, C., Grgic, J., & Lara, B. (2019). The influence of the menstrual cycle on muscle strength and power performance. *Journal of Human Kinetics, 68*, 123–133. https://doi.org/10.2478/hukin-2019-0061

Rootd. (2023, April 30). The debate over natural vs. synthetic vitamins: What you need to know. https://rootd.com/blogs/vitamins-minerals-101/the-debate-over-natural-vs-synthetic-vitamins-what-you-need-to-know

Rupa Health. (n.d.). Thyroid. https://www.rupahealth.com/health-categories/thyroid

Sangalli, C. N., Leffa, P. d.S., de Morais, M. B., & Vitolo, M. R. (2018). Infant feeding practices and the effect in reducing functional constipation 6 years later: A randomized field trial. *Journal of Pediatric Gastroenterology and Nutrition, 67*(5), 584–590. https://doi.org/10.1097/MPG.0000000000002075

Sharma, R. D., Raghuram, T. C., & Rao, N. S. (1990). Effect of fenugreek seeds on blood glucose and serum lipids in type I diabetes. *European Journal of Clinical Nutrition, 44*(4), 301–306.

Shimizu, M. (2012). Modulation of intestinal functions by dietary substances: An effective approach to health promotion. *Journal of Traditional and Complementary Medicine, 2*(2), 81–83. https://doi.org/10.1016/s2225-4110(16)30080-3

Shulhai, A. M., Rotondo, R., Petraroli, M., Patianna, V., Predieri, B., Iughetti, L., Esposito, S., & Street, M. E. (2024). The role of nutrition on thyroid function. *Nutrients, 16*(15), 2496. https://doi.org/10.3390/nu16152496

Sidhu, S. R. K., Kok, C. W., Kunasegaran, T., & Ramadas, A. (2023). Effect of plant-based diets on gut microbiota: A systematic review of interventional studies. *Nutrients, 15*(6), 1510. https://doi.org/10.3390/nu15061510

Siminiuc, R., & Ţurcanu, D. (2023). Impact of nutritional diet therapy on premenstrual syndrome. *Frontiers in Nutrition, 10,* 1079417. https://doi.org/10.3389/fnut.2023.1079417

Singh, R. P., & Bhardwaj, A. (2023). β-glucans: A potential source for maintaining gut microbiota and the immune system. *Frontiers in Nutrition, 10,* 1143682. https://doi.org/10.3389/fnut.2023.1143682

Soliman, G. A. (2019). Dietary fiber, atherosclerosis, and cardiovascular disease. *Nutrients, 11*(5), 1155. https://doi.org/10.3390/nu11051155

Stohs, S. J. (2014). Safety and efficacy of shilajit (mumie, moomiyo). *Phytotherapy Research: PTR, 28*(4), 475–479. https://doi.org/10.1002/ptr.5018

Taghizadeh, M., Farzin, N., Taheri, S., Mahlouji, M., Akbari, H., Karamali, F., & Asemi, Z. (2017). The effect of dietary supplements containing green tea, capsaicin, and ginger extracts on weight loss and metabolic profiles in overweight women: A randomized double-blind placebo-controlled clinical trial. *Annals of Nutrition and Metabolism, 70*(4), 277–285. https://doi.org/10.1159/000471889

Tallei, T. E., Fatimawali, N. J., Idroes, R., Zidan, B. M. R. M., Mitra, S., Celik, I., Nainu, F., Ağagündüz, D., Emran, T. B., & Capasso, R. (2021). A comprehensive review of the potential use of green tea polyphenols in the management of COVID-19. *Evidence-Based Complementary and Alternative Medicine: eCAM, 2021,* 7170736. https://doi.org/10.1155/2021/7170736

van Vliet, S., Burd, N. A., & van Loon, L. J. (2015). The skeletal muscle anabolic response to plant- versus animal-based protein consumption. *The Journal of Nutrition, 145*(9), 1981–1991. https://doi.org/10.3945/jn.114.204305

Vilaplana-Pérez, C., Auñón, D., García-Flores, L. A., & Gil-Izquierdo, A. (2014). Hydroxytyrosol and potential uses in cardiovascular diseases, cancer, and AIDS. *Frontiers in Nutrition, 1,* 18. https://doi.org/10.3389/fnut.2014.00018

Vinderola, G., Cotter, P. D., Freitas, M., Gueimonde, M., Holscher, H. D., Ruas-Madiedo, P., Salminen, S., Swanson, K. S., Sanders, M. E., & Cifelli, C. J. (2023). Fermented foods: A perspective on their role in delivering biotics. *Frontiers in Microbiology, 14,* article 1196239. https://doi.org/10.3389/fmicb.2023.1196239

Wahab, S., Annadurai, S., Abullais, S. S., Das, G., Ahmad, W., Ahmad, M. F., Kandasamy, G., Vasudevan, R., Ali, M. S., & Amir, M. (2021). Glycyrrhiza glabra (Licorice): A comprehensive review on its phytochemistry, biological activities, clinical evidence and toxicology. *Plants (Basel, Switzerland), 10*(12), 2751. https://doi.org/10.3390/plants10122751

Wahl, D. R., Villinger, K., König, L. M., Ziesemer, K., Schupp, H. T., & Renner, B. (2017). Healthy food choices are happy food choices: Evidence from a real life sample using smartphone based assessments. *Scientific Reports, 7*(1), 17069. https://doi.org/10.1038/s41598-017-17262-9

Wallace, T. C., Murray, R., & Zelman, K. M. (2016). The nutritional value and health benefits of chickpeas and hummus. *Nutrients, 8*(12), 766. https://doi.org/10.3390/nu8120766

Wang, X., Qi, Y., & Zheng, H. (2022). Dietary polyphenol, gut microbiota, and health benefits. *Antioxidants (Basel, Switzerland), 11*(6), 1212. https://doi.org/10.3390/antiox11061212

Wang, Y., Yao, X., Shen, H., Zhao, R., Li, Z., Shen, X., Wang, F., Chen, K., Zhou, Y., Li, B., Zheng, X., & Lu, S. (2022). Nutritional composition, efficacy, and processing of Vigna angularis (adzuki bean) for the human diet: An overview. *Molecules (Basel, Switzerland), 27*(18), 6079. https://doi.org/10.3390/molecules27186079

Wani, A. L., Bhat, S. A., & Ara, A. (2015). Omega-3 fatty acids and the treatment of depression: A review of scientific evidence. *Integrative Medicine Research, 4*(3), 132–141. https://doi.org/10.1016/j.imr.2015.07.003

Ware, M. (2023, November 29). Is edamame good for you? Nutrition, calories, recipes, benefits, and all you need to know. *Medical News Today.* https://www.medicalnewstoday.com/articles/280285#nutrition

Weaver, J. (2021, July 12). Fermented-food diet increases microbiome diversity, decreases inflammatory proteins, study finds. Stanford Medicine News Center. https://med.stanford.edu/news/all-news/2021/07/fermented-food-diet-increases-microbiome-diversity-lowers-inflammation

WebMD. (2023, June 5). Difference between wild and farm-raised salmon. https://www.webmd.com/diet/difference-between-wild-and-farmed-salmon

———. (2024, September 24). Foods high in zinc. https://www.webmd.com/diet/foods-high-in-zinc

Weizmann Institute of Science. (2015, November 19). Blood sugar levels in response to foods are highly individual. Weizmann Wonder Wander. https://wis-wander.weizmann.ac.il/life-sciences/blood-sugar-levels-response-foods-are-highly-individual

Wiertsema, S. P., van Bergenhenegouwen, J., Garssen, J., & Knippels, L. M. J. (2021). The interplay between the gut microbiome and the immune system in the context of infectious diseases throughout life and the role of nutrition in optimizing treatment strategies. *Nutrients, 13*(3), 886. https://doi.org/10.3390/nu13030886

Wilding, J. P. H., Batterham, R. L., Calanna, S., Davies, M., Van Gaal, L. F., Lingvay, I., McGowan, B. M., Rosenstock, J., Tran, M. T.

D., Wadden, T. A., Wharton, S., Yokote, K., Zeuthen, N., Kushner, R. F., & STEP 1 Study Group. (2021). Once-weekly semaglutide in adults with overweight or obesity. *The New England Journal of Medicine, 384*(11), 989–1002. https://doi.org/10.1056/NEJMoa2032183

Wolfe, R. R. (2017). Branched-chain amino acids and muscle protein synthesis in humans: Myth or reality? *Journal of the International Society of Sports Nutrition, (14)*30. https://doi.org/10.1186/s12970-017-0184-9

Wu, X., Qian, L., Liu, K., Wu, J., & Shan, Z. (2021). Gastrointestinal microbiome and gluten in celiac disease. *Annals of Medicine, 53*(1), 1797–1805. https://doi.org/10.1080/07853890.2021.1990392

Wyatt, K. M., Dimmock, P. W., Jones, P. W., & Shaughn O'Brien, P. M. (1999). Efficacy of vitamin B6 in the treatment of premenstrual syndrome: Systematic review. *BMJ (Clinical research ed.), 318*(7195), 1375–1381. https://doi.org/10.1136/bmj.318.7195.1375

Yang, M., & Wang, Y. (2022). Recent advances and the mechanism of astaxanthin in ophthalmological diseases. *Journal of Ophthalmology, 2022,* 8071406. https://doi.org/10.1155/2022/8071406

Yi, X., & Muha, C. (2022, May 22). Gut dysbiosis has the potential to reduce the sexual attractiveness of mouse female. *Frontiers in Microbiology, 13.* https://doi.org/10.3389/fmicb.2022.916766

Yin, J., Li, Y., Li, X., Li, L., & Zhang, J. (2008). Efficacy of berberine in patients with type 2 diabetes mellitus. *Metabolism: Clinical and Experimental, 57*(5), 712–717. https://doi.org/10.1016/j.metabol.2007.12.010

Yoshino, J., Baur, J. A., & Imai, S. I. (2018). NAD+ intermediates: The biology and therapeutic potential of NMN and NR. *Cell Metabolism, 27*(3), 513–528. https://doi.org/10.1016/j.cmet.2017.11.002

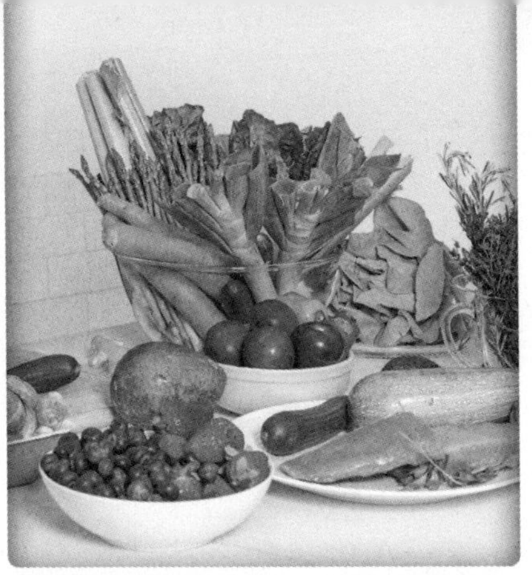

About the Author

Ella Davar, RD, is an internationally recognized dietitian, speaker, and longevity expert specializing in gut health and personalized nutrition. Based in Miami, she is also a certified holistic health coach, yoga and meditation teacher, and the creator of The Gut-Brain Method™, a pioneering course that integrates microbiome science with mindfulness techniques to optimize digestion, mental health, and longevity. Over the past decade, she has empowered thousands of clients worldwide to achieve sustainable health and metabolic resilience through an integrative, science-backed approach.

Ella's expertise has been featured across leading media outlets, including *MindBodyGreen, Forbes, People, Shape,* and *Women's Health,* and she is a regular guest on television in South Florida and New York. She frequently speaks at high-profile wellness events and hosts longevity-focused retreats and dinners at top venues worldwide, including Miami's #1 wellness resort, The Carillon Hotel.